PREVENTING ALZHEIMER'S AND OTHER DEMENTIAS

Barry K. Spiker, PhD
Eliot Jekowsky, PhD, MD
Colleen Hunsaker, DO

Kitty Kat Press™

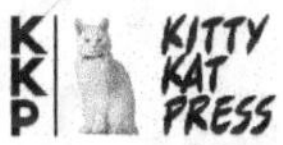

Copyright © 2020 Barry K. Spiker, PhD

Published by: Kitty Kat Press™

Kitty Kat Press™
Visit our website: https://kittykatpress.com

Artwork by Mary Linda Mills

Buy the Kindle eBook to use the hyperlinks

Printed in the United States of America

CONTENTS

HOW TO USE THIS BOOK

Preventing Alzheimer's and Other Dementias NOW is an eBook (electronic book) that takes advantage of the rich content of the internet. It allows the reader to jump to a selected section of the book, click on a hyperlink to go to an article or articles in an internet search domain, and then toggle back to the eBook.

This eBook has been reviewed extensively and feedback has been instrumental in helping us understand how people approach and use it. We have received extremely positive comments on readers' ability to fully engage with the material. We were told by several esteemed neurologists that this book is the best compendium of the best research currently available; that this book can help you become more health-literate; and that this book can facilitate a better conversation between care-givers, health professionals and patients. We hope you will use it often.

Preventing Alzheimer's and Other Dementias NOW can be read without an internet connection to get a solid overview of the **BEEMS** model for mitigating cognitive decline. When connected to the Internet, links allow readers to access primary sources and other stories, studies, papers, videos, books, pictures, and multimedia related to a citation.

To assist the user with navigation, Table of Contents (ToC) entries are linked to corresponding sections in the eBook. Additionally, each page contains a link that will take the user back to the ToC.

Each boxed item in this eBook is a link to a Google Search Results Page that lists items relevant to the topic. The resource specified in the boxed item that was selected will be included in this list. Additionally, because the search results page also contains an extensive list of other relevant items, the reader may browse these results for articles, videos, images, and recent news articles that may be of interest.

As stated above, each boxed hyperlink takes the user to a Google Search Results Page where the target reference will be found. However, should the user instead wish to directly access the target article or study, the link contained in the Listing of Sources found at the back of the eBook will take the user directly to the target.

If this eBook is read on a tablet or smartphone, then the reader will need to toggle between the eBook and the Google Search Results page. If the eBook is accessed in anything but a web browser, then the <back> button will not return the reader to the eBook, but will go to the Table of Contents (ToC).

 We want you to enjoy this eBook as much as we enjoyed writing it.

PREFACE

Every 3 seconds, someone is diagnosed with dementia somewhere around the globe. Currently 50 million people have dementia and, according to Alzheimer's Disease International, by the year 2050, 150 million people will have been diagnosed. We can and must respond to this growing epidemic.

On July 14, 2019, the American Alzheimer's International Conference came out with the following press release which states that changing lifestyle choices could help prevent dementia. Now this eBook says the same.

> **Lifestyle Interventions Provide Maximum Memory Benefit When Combined, May Offset Elevated Alzheimer's Risk Due to Genetics, Pollution**

The purpose of this book is to provide the reader with the best education available on how to mitigate or slow cognitive decline, followed by presentation of a framework to support personal action planning. In slightly more than 100 pages, we have curated and summarized the latest evidence on lifestyle and behavioral changes that can affect cognitive decline.

Preventing Alzheimer's and Other Dementias NOW provides summaries of the evidence-based, holistic, and non-invasive research for scientists and practicing medical professionals; and provides overviews of readable, intelligible articles for the everyday reader. It is a meta-synthesis of the best research on individual interventions that have been shown to slow down the onset of cognitive decline that may come with aging. We believe that Alzheimer's and other dementia's might be preventable or, at least slowed. We came to that belief that after reading thousands of studies over the past 10 years and summarizing for you the best and most impactful of those studies.

Our conclusions were recently backed up by the launch of "The Lancet's" Commission Dementia Prevention, Intervention and Care in July of 2017. Much of what has been reported by "The Lancet" was known earlier and this eBook highlights that specific research. To have written a book that is largely backed up by what "The Lancet" reports is both confirming and humbling. This nearly two hundred year old family of journals is considered one of the most prestigious journals in the fields of science and medicine. It exists at its core as a journal that believes that medicine must serve society and provide knowledge that must transform society and must lead to improving lives. And, that is why we wanted to write this book-in order to improve the lives of anyone who might suffer the effects of Alzheimer's and other dementias.

The Lancet's Commission and Report

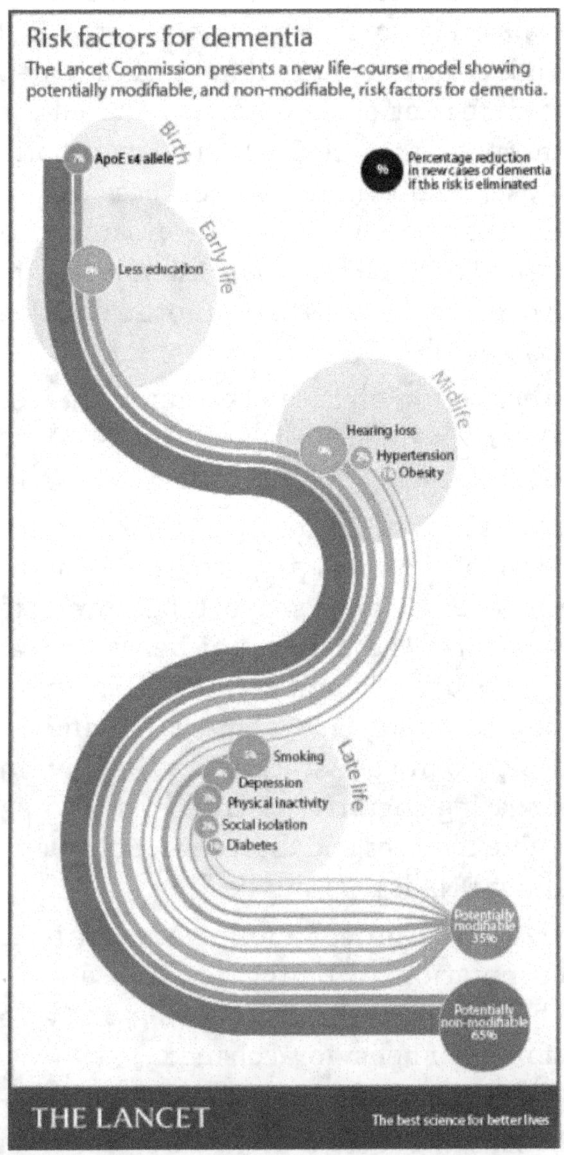

This eBook begins with a Background section that includes definitions of Alzheimer's and related cognitive disorders, a description of how environment can impact health, a discussion of personal costs related to these disorders, and an overview of the emerging focus on epigenetics.

The book continues with a discussion of the best medical research available on factors that have the potential to mitigate cognitive decline. Included are hundreds of hyperlinks to related, indepth information. Collectively, the authors have over 135 total years of work experience and have published dozens of studies, books, chapters, and articles. Based on their reviews, the best medical research available from around the world is presented here. These findings are intended to position the reader to make better choices to promote a healthier brain and a higher quality of life

Included in the section on the most important studies are the China Study, Braak's Hypothesis, the Nun Study, the PreDIVA Study, the FINGER Study, MAPT RCT, and the POINTER Study.

Following the research section, the **BEEMS** protocol is presented in detail. The **BEEMS** protocol has been developed by the Epigenesis Corporation to support individual efforts to take action and optimize the benefits of behavioral and lifestyle changes that have been demonstrated by research. The **BEEMS** protocol (Body, Emotion, Environment, Mindfulness, and Spirituality) is designed in a holistic and non-invasive manner with a goal of mitigating cognitive decline and fending off associated diagnosable diseases and disorders. Epigenetics holds the promise that our DNA is NOT our destiny.

Detail on the **BEEMS** protocol is followed by an introduction to Epigenesis Corporation, including its purpose, a description of its focus on health and wellness coaching, and an overview of various platforms for behavioral change.

Final sections bring to light the impact of dementia on organizations, including costs; and the caregiver crisis, including the impact on individuals of taking on caregiver responsibilities. This final section includes an important discussion on caregiving and caregivers, and identifies resources that support individuals providing critical care to those suffering from these debilitating diseases.

There may never be cures for dementia or Alzheimer's Disease as there are for other devastating diseases such as some types of cancer and heart disease. However, we believe there is a viable approach, through awareness and prevention, to take care of ourselves before any deleterious changes begin to happen in our brains and our bodies. By remaining healthy throughout our lives, we maximize the potential of delaying or offsetting cognitive decline, and preventing our brains from facing an uncertain and catastrophic future. This eBook was written to help people take responsibility for their health and wellness and embrace the possibilities for healing before becoming ill.

This book was written from a place of love and hope, not fear.

The contents of this eBook, along with the information represented by the hundreds of links contained herein, represent a massive encyclopedic reference document. We believe that this is the most current, valid and definitive resource for anyone interested in studying or understanding cognitive decline and its associated disorders or diseases, prevention methods, and the current state of published research about dementia. We fervently believe this book will increase your health literacy and help families and caregivers have more fruitful conversations with their primary care physicians, specialists or caregivers.

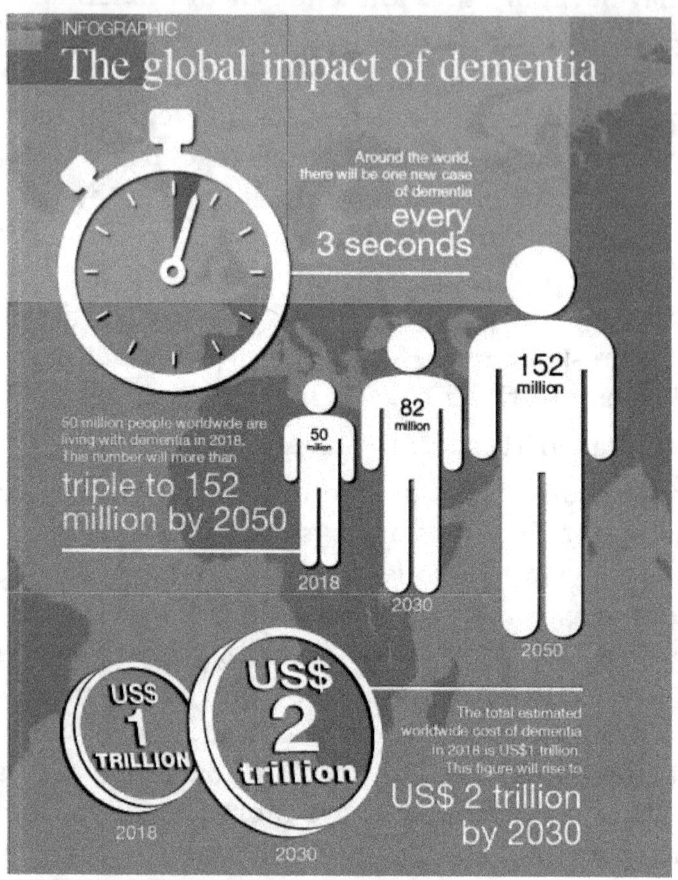

World Alzheimer Report 2018

INTRODUCTION

Ten or more years ago (or, even now) the words "you have can-cer" might be the worst words you could ever hear from your family doctor.

Today, many cancers are curable and treatable. We believe that the most dreadful medical diagnosis that you could hear today is "you have dementia." These words are likely a death sentence that can stretch over many years and will negatively influence and change families, communities, and the financial futures of everyone impacted by this disease. Dementia is near pandemic proportions in Japan, the country with the world's most elderly population, and is growing exponentially around the world, especially in the poorest of countries.

In the past decade in the United States, we have seen a large and growing epidemic of Alzheimer's with an 87% rise in its prevalence and mortality in the last ten years. It is only going to get worse.

> **2019 Alzheimer's Disease Facts and Figures**

We are living longer on average, and this means that increasing numbers of people will endure some form of cognitive decline in the later stages of life. In its severest form, cognitive decline results in a range of diseases that most often takes the form of dementia. As our population ages, most of us will be affected, either directly or indirectly, by this current epidemic.

Researchers, the business community, governments, the public, and other stakeholders are seeking ways to extend our lives.

But we ask the question, what good is it to be alive at 100 years old when in the last 20 years of life, you are suffering from dementia?

Types of Dementia

To further complicate the issue, research shows that medical diagnostics are fallible in determining the root causes of disorders. There is ample evidence that medical testing can lead medical professionals to incorrectly qualify an individual as prone to specific diseases. Statistically, many individuals do not and will never suffer from cognitive decline and dementia, despite their genetic profile.

Likewise, even if every person were to do everything indicated as promising by scientific research, some might still suffer from dementia. Despite having no definitive precursors, there will be those who succumb to these diseases. This precise predicament leads us to propose the BEEMS protocol to mitigate the risk of cognitive decline associated with aging.

BEEMS is the Epigenesis Corporation's systems approach and methodology designed to mitigate the severity of cognitive decline. It capitalizes on the best known research and studies in the areas of beneficial lifestyle and behavioral factors like diet, exercise, mindfulness and a higher power.

The Epigenesis Corporation offers not only a systems approach to evaluating risk factors and identifying appropriate action, but it also offers behavioral coaching to support the individual in their efforts to make positive changes, thereby increasing the likelihood of successful change.

Additional research and scientific study will demonstrate the efficacy of our interventions in mitigation efforts. Much more scientific due diligence is needed to actualize the realistic gains from implementing the **BEEMS** framework.

Governments, hospitals, insurance companies, and donors will need to invest billions into additional research to test the efficacy of specific therapies. We are confident that this research will eventually conclude that an epigenetic approach that invokes "cellular memory" is most effective at combating cognitive decline.

Acute injuries require specific measures to fix them, heal them, and rehabilitate them. An epigenetic approach starts with preventive care, knowing your own healthcare needs, and knowing what must change. When a personalized, integrative, holistic, evidence-based, and functional approach to health is adopted, individuals will realize wellness through healthy behaviors.

We have brought together some of the best health and wellness coaches who just happen to all have advanced degrees and certifications and nearly 30 years of experience helping people with changing their behaviors. We bring together nutritionists, sports therapists, medical doctors and many specialists to augment your experience with your lead coach. Please reach out to Barry at b.spiker@att.net or call 480-721-7308 or visit our website at http://www.epigenesiscorp.com to get started.

Remember, you have a right to be an individual as well as an obligation (with thanks to Eleanor Roosevelt). The choices we make are our own responsibility and we must make them well.

We want to say, here's to your health, wellness and longevity!

Live long and prosper as Spock would say.

The World Health Organization (WHO) designed the following two posters to help people better understand the public health priority of dementia. It starts with a brief overview of symptoms of dementia. Who is affected, what does it cost and a somewhat abbreviated expression of the causes of dementia. Our book delves into all the topics much more deeply.

Then, the WHO shows you their action plan and some excellent targets for change. Please examine all of them. Make yourself part of the solution and see how you can become involved in your local community.

Dementia from the Perspective of the World Health Organization

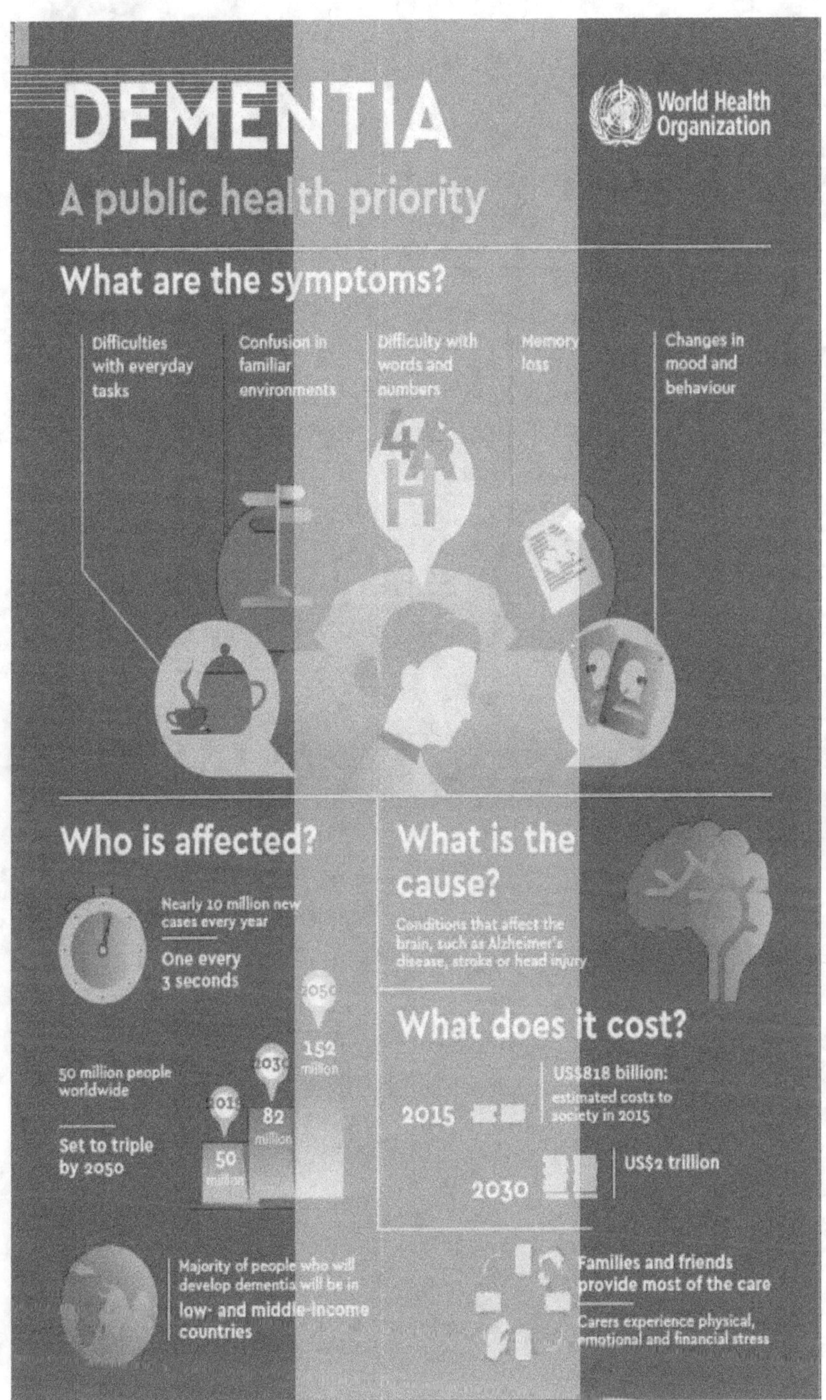
DEMENTIA
A public health priority
World Health Organization

What are the symptoms?

Difficulties with everyday tasks
Confusion in familiar environments
Difficulty with words and numbers
Memory loss
Changes in mood and behaviour

Who is affected?

Nearly 10 million new cases every year
One every 3 seconds
50 million people worldwide
Set to triple by 2050

2050
152 million
2030
82 million
2018
50 million

What is the cause?
Conditions that affect the brain, such as Alzheimer's disease, stroke or head injury

What does it cost?

2015
US$818 billion: estimated costs to society in 2015

2030
US$2 trillion

Majority of people who will develop dementia will be in low- and middle-income countries

Families and friends provide most of the care
Carers experience physical, emotional and financial stress

The Global Action Plan on the Public Health Response to Dementia 2017 - 2025

Vision

A world in which dementia is prevented and people with dementia and their carers live well and receive the care and support they need to fulfil their potential with dignity, respect, autonomy and equality.

Goal

To improve the lives of people with dementia, their carers and families, while decreasing the impact of dementia on them as well as on communities and countries.

The seven action areas and targets

Dementia as a public health priority

Dementia awareness and friendliness

Dementia risk reduction

Dementia diagnosis, treatment & care

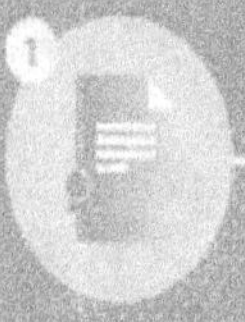

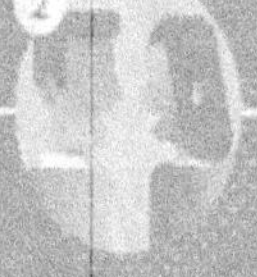

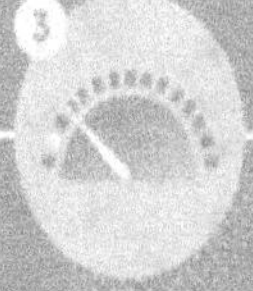

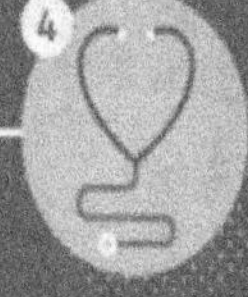

By 2025, 75% of countries have national policies, strategies, plans or frameworks for dementia

By 2025, 100% of countries have a functioning public-awareness campaign on dementia

By 2025, 50% of countries have at least one dementia-friendly initiative

Risk reduction targets identified in the Global action plan for prevention and control of noncommunicable diseases 2013-2020 are achieved

By 2025, 50% of people with dementia are diagnosed, in at least 50% of countries

Support for dementia carers

Information systems for dementia

Dementia research and innovation

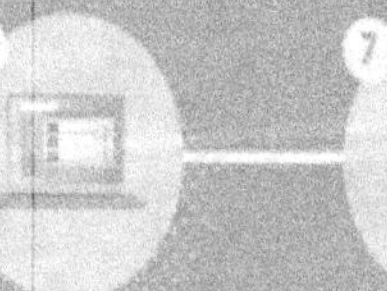

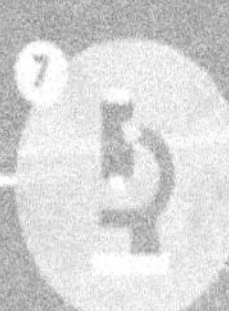

By 2025, 75% of countries provide support and training for carers and families

By 2025, 50% of countries routinely collect data on core dementia indicators

Global research output on dementia doubles between 2017 and 2025

BACKGROUND

INFLUENCE OF THE ENVIRONMENT

Environmental factors can be drivers for the modification of gene expression–what we call epigenetics. Over a lifetime, the emotional, personal, and physical characteristics of daily life can dramatically influence health. For example, we now understand that traumatic stress and other environmental influences in early childhood can leave a child vulnerable to many physical health issues, learning difficulties, and mental distress. Behaviors such as smoking tobacco can affect the onset of lung disease and dementia regardless of the degree of genetic predisposition. Even growing up in nature, living a productive and happy life and eating well can leave you susceptible to unsuspected environmental influences. Toxicity from the environment can be introduced from anywhere and can dramatically affect health and well-being.

> ## Dementia from Toxic Substances

Chronic inflammation is also associated with dementia and can begin in childhood. The inflammation pathway is problematic for all kinds of chronic illnesses and is not often measured or diagnosed in a typical annual physical exam.

> ## Chronic Inflammation Linked to Dementia

Inflammation in mid-life, e.g., in the 40s or 50s, can be associated with dementia. Inflammation earlier in life may also start the process. By the time inflammation is discovered, it may be too late, as the brain may already have started shrinking.

Could Inflammation in Midlife Predict Dementia?

The level of white matter in the brain may also be something to focus on if an MRI taken during middle age shows an increase. C Reactive Protein (CRP, the white matter) is a measure of inflammation.

Shades of White: Diffusion Properties of T1-and FLAIR-defined White Matter Signal Abnormalities Differ in Stages from Cognitively Normal to Dementia

The Association of Mid-to Late-Life Systemic Inflammation with White Matter Structure in Older Adults. The Atherosclerosis Risk in Communities Study

The impact of depletion of gut bacteria in recent studies signals another promising approach to studying dementia. Later we will examine Braak's Hypothesis as a significant, early finding for Parkinson's Disease, another form of dementia. In 2003, the German neuropathologist Heiko Braak presented a theory suggesting that Parkinson's disease begins in the gut and spreads to the brain. Also, the notion that the sense of smell is an indicator of Parkinson's begins with this hypothesis. Future studies will continue to examine the association between the gut microbiome and dementia.

Dementia and Gut Bacteria: New Research Shows Link

More current research connecting food and digestion with brain health is available in the **BEEMS** section on Diet. In that section we further explore the critical role of the gut micro-biome.

Effect of Probiotic Supplementation on Cognitive Function and Metabolic Status in Alzheimer's Disease: A Randomized, Double-Blind and Controlled Trial

The connection between the gut and the brain should be better understood by both laymen and the medical community. The gut-brain connection refers to the physical and chemical connections between these major systems of the body. What you eat can affect your brain health. Research on the vagus nerve, which interfaces with the parasympathetic control of the heart, lungs, and gut, shows us part of the reason.

The Gut-Brain Connection: How it Works and the Role of Nutrition

The linkage of the gut-brain microbiome is further explained in the article below, which offers new approaches for the study of Parkinson's.

A Gut-Brain Link for Parkinson's Gets a Closer Look

Potential healthful interventions that science did not consider heretofore continue to be explored. What is truly exciting is that the key results of current research on what are considered preventable forms of dementia are now being made available to us all, and are contained in this book.

Prevalence of Treatable and Reversible Dementias:

A Study in a Dementia Outpatient Clinic

An excellent summary of dementia, its causes and symptoms, and possibly preventable forms of dementia appears on the Mayo Clinic website.

Dementia Describes a Group of Symptoms Affecting Memory, Thinking, and Social Abilities...

MORE ON ALZHEIMER'S, DEMENTIA, AND COGNITIVE DECLINE

Alzheimer's disease is a form of mental deterioration that can start in middle age or old age and becomes progressively more debilitating. Dementia is a general term for a decline in mental abilities severe enough to interfere with daily life. Cognitive decline may occur with aging, but aging is not always a precursor to dementia. Alzheimer's is probably the best-known form of dementia. It is important to understand the differences between age-related cognitive decline and various forms of dementia.

In 2017, the National Academy of Sciences, Engineering, and Medicine summarized findings from funded research studies focused on the mitigation of cognitive decline and dementia. In the report, three broad types of cognitive decline and dementia were defined:

- Age-related cognitive decline,
- Mild cognitive impairment, and
- Dementias (including Clinically Defined Alzheimer's Disease (CDAD)).

The National Institute on Aging defines several major types of dementias such as Clinical Alzheimer's disease, Frontotemporal disorders, and Lewy body dementia. People can have more than one of these dementias and dementia-like conditions. These are considered "mixed dementia."

What Is Mixed Dementia?

As clinically defined, Alzheimer's disease is difficult to definitively diagnose, and mixed forms are perhaps even more difficult to identify. For example, Alzheimer's and other dementias often co-occur with vascular disease, that is, they are comorbidities. Some patients have both vascular-related impairments and vascular dementia.

TDP-43 Stage, Mixed Pathologies, and Clinical Alzheimer's-type Dementia

LONG-TERM PERSONAL AND FINANCIAL COSTS

A profound sense of urgency should be internalized by every American and by all of us as global citizens. Those in charge of running organizations and determining public policy need to address long-term costs. Harry Johns, President and CEO of the U.S. Alzheimer's Association, stated before a subcommittee of the Committee on Appropriations, United States House of Representatives in 2013, that "...the graying of America threatens the bankrupting of America."

> **Testimony of Harry Johns, President and CEO of the Alzheimer's Association**

Costs vary, but overall, "caring for people with Alzheimer's will cost all payers – Medicare, Medicaid and private insurance – over $20 trillion over the next 40 years." If this report does not wake everyone up to the urgent need to address this problem, perhaps nothing will.

A story aired by *CBS News 60 Minutes* takes the current situation to a personal level and demonstrates the urgency of considering these issues. It describes the journey of one family and its impacts on their lives.

"For ten years, Dr. Jon LaPook has been checking in on Carol Daly, a woman diagnosed with Alzheimer's, and her caregiver husband, Mike. After a decade, the disease has had a devastating impact on each of them." This is truly a story about "for better or for worse" – tragic yet compelling.

> ## Following a Couple from Diagnosis to the Final Stages of Alzheimer's

Stories like the Daly's make a case for health professionals and financial planners to help disseminate information earlier and more thoroughly. Professionals, including legal, financial, social, medical, and psychological professionals, all need training on the implications of dementia. Researchers and institutions responsible for training these professionals also should commit to obtaining a much better understanding of the impacts of aging.

It is vital that professionals inform the general population of what the future may hold and what steps may help mitigate impact.

One place to turn for help with financial impact is the community of Financial Gerontologists. The American Institute of Financial Gerontology conducts corporate training in Financial Gerontology for professionals in finance and provides counsel to older consumers and their families.

> ## American Institute of Financial Gerontology

Bank of America and other corporations are taking notice. They are beginning to be proactive in addressing the graying of America.

> ## Bank of America Merrill Lynch's Director of Financial Gerontology Cyndi Hutchins Named Influencer in Aging by PBS's Next Avenue

Private sector leaders have initiated the CEOi, which initially advocated for finding a cure for Alzheimer's by 2020. Of course, now we are well into 2020 and there is still no cure.

> **Us Against Alzheimer's**

Other organizations such as Next Avenue are dedicated to being news aggregators for people over 50 (they are part of PBS). Next Avenue has a great product and service.

> **Next Avenue**

Earlier we cited the National Academies of Sciences, Engineering, and Medicine, who reported that although there are distinctions between cognitive decline and various dementias, common symptoms of these disorders may be mitigated with similar interventions, including lifestyle changes. All forms of dementia are challenging to treat effectively, but newly emerging science provides us with pathways and alternatives to consider.

There have been many claims in the media and in research findings that support interventions that may delay or mitigate the disease. Available medical research that is presented here makes the case for individual interventions as well as the use of collective, holistic interventions to mitigate severity of cognitive decline and dementia. When the evidence is viewed critically, there is still much to learn and understand, but in the meantime, personal interventions may be adopted by individuals NOW.

The question becomes, can we afford to wait to make changes if there are things we can do now, on our own? The reasons we should take steps to delay or mitigate symptoms are apparent and are prominently reported in the following article, "The

Value of Delaying Alzheimer's Disease Onset."

The Value of Delaying Alzheimer's Disease Onset

All forms of Alzheimer's are ultimately devastating for families. These diseases often begin at later stages in a person's life, but early-onset Alzheimer's is also reaching epidemic proportions.

Early and Late-Onset Alzheimer's Disease: What Are the Differences?

Late-Onset Alzheimer's Disease (LOAD) has a distinctly different genetic origin than early-onset Alzheimer's. However, it is striking that not everyone who has a known genetic or heritable predisposition toward Alzheimer's disease, other dementias, or cognitive decline will develop one of these diseases. In response to this phenomenon, researchers are using the new discipline of epigenetics to better understand the impacts of our behaviors and external environment on cells, genes, disease, and health. More on this in the next section.

Comorbidities are diagnoses like high blood pressure, vascular disease, and diabetes that can co-occur with Alzheimer's and impact patient outcomes. Comorbidities make treating forms of dementia more costly, complicated, confusing, and potentially error-prone. Given all the costs and devastating outcomes of Alzheimer's, dementia and associated comorbidities, it is promising that there is an official pronouncement from the U.S. government on possibilities for prevention. This statement is included in the following information from the Agency for Healthcare Research and Quality.

Comorbidity and Progression of Late-Onset Alzheimer's Disease: A Systematic Review

Non-Psychiatric Comorbidity Associated

with Alzheimer's Disease
Alzheimer's Disease Associated with Psychiatric Comorbidities
Alzheimer's Epidemic Hits Women Hardest

PREVENTION AND THE NEW FOCUS ON EPIGENETICS

Through the Agency for Healthcare Research and Quality's (AHRQ) Evidence-based Practices Center, the Department of Health and Human Services published a report reviewing the research results and strength of evidence for specific interventions to deter cognitive decline, mild cognitive impairment, and clinical-type Alzheimer's dementia.

> **Preventing Cognitive Decline and Dementia: A Way Forward**

The science is not *settled*, but the interest among researchers remains high, and the publication of research articles in this area has grown in the last ten years such that evaluation of the strength of results has become more viable. Although much of the research on these topics is still in its infancy, some suggested practical information is making its way to the public.

> **Interventions to Prevent Age-Related Cognitive Decline, Mild Cognitive Impairment, and Clinical Alzheimer's-Type Dementia**

None of the interventions discussed in the following reference were found to produce what the agency termed as "strong evidence" for the efficacy of specific mitigation efforts. The AHRQ did, however, find some support for the notion that cognitive training may improve memory temporarily for participants without progressed cognitive impairment. Another finding was that there is little or weak evidence that any such interventions are effective for those diagnosed with clinical Alzheimer's. The indications overall were that physical exercise and vitamin B12 plus folic acid are promising avenues to pursue in attempts to mitigate the symptoms of more serious cognitive decline.

These results are consistent with the findings of the National Institute of Aging website mentioned in the Introduction. Other recent reviews support the claim that physical exercise is essential. These reviews are available in the section under our discussion of Body.

> ## Not Much Can Prevent Alzheimer's, but 3 Common Practices May Help

Findings of original research papers are included in this eBook, and we will walk through those. To continue to build familiarity with research results written for the everyday consumer, see a recent article in *Parade* magazine entitled "The Cheater's Guide to Beating Alzheimer's."

This citation includes some information on the genetics of Alzheimer's as well as a summary of interventions.

> ## The Cheater's Guide to Beating Alzheimer's: New Research and Prevention Breakthroughs

Research backs up our belief that if an individual practices the BEEMS protocol, builds a behavioral platform through epigenetics, and uses a behavioral coach to set goals and reach milestones, better health and well-being will result.

> ## Nine Lifestyle Changes Can Reduce
> ## Dementia Risk, Study Says

Epigenetics

> ### Epigenetics: The Panacea for Cognitive Decline?

Epigenetics literally means "above" or "on top of" genetics, and dates back to Aristotle. It is a term used to suggest that it is not only genes that make us who we are. Scientists define epigenetics as the study of changes in organisms initiated by modification of *gene expression* rather than by changes in genetic structure or code. In other words, a change in gene structure or mutation need not occur to realize a change in how a gene may function.

> ## The Public Reception of Putative
> ## Epigenetic Mechanisms in the
> ## Transgenerational Effects of Trauma

The epigenome is the "software" which gives instructions to our "hardware" (our DNA). As the term 'epigenetics' makes its way into the popular lexicon, more and more people are coming to realize that we are complicated biological creatures that need opportunities to shine despite our "hardware."

The epigenetic intention is to build what is called "molecular memory." These are habits and behaviors learned through positive interventions that can mitigate cognitive decline and hence dementia. Genes can remember the steps you take to make yourself stronger, healthier, more aware, and more alive. While we will not get into the "weeds" of this form of "epi-memory" by discussing methyl groups, histones and DNA methylation, suffice it to say that researchers have just begun to study this phenomenon, and after nearly sixty thousand research articles, epigenetics is starting to be understood by a broader audience.

> ## Muscles 'Remember' Previous Exercise in the Form of Epigenetic Tags on DNA

We find a similar phenomenon with nutrition as with muscular research. As the abstract of the following paper says, "Human and experimental animal studies have highlighted the link between alterations in the early life environment and increased risk of obesity and metabolic disorders in later life." The somewhat radical notion is that what your mother ate while you were in the womb can have an impact on your health later in life. Just as periods of muscle growth are remembered by the genes in your muscles, your epigenome accounts for the state of your genes during previous periods in your life.

> ## Early Life Nutrition, Epigenetics, and Programming of Later Life Disease

> ## Maternal Diet May Program Child for Disease Risk, but Better Nutrition Later Can Change That

Epigenetics is an ontology that includes linking developmental exposures to long-term toxicity, and is a powerful explanation of our nature as human beings.

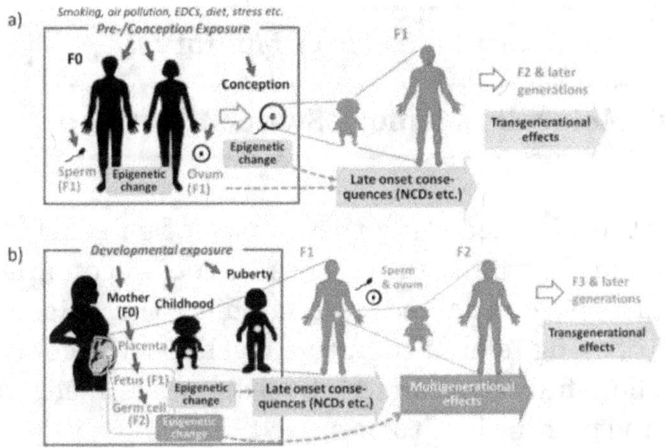

Epigenetics as a Mechanism Linking Developmental Exposures to Long-Term Toxicity

Epigenetic changes caused by developmental environmental exposures are implicated in long-term/late-onset health effects. Development is vulnerable to environmental insults. The critical periods include (a) pre-conception and conception, and (b) in utero, childhood and puberty. Epigenetic alterations, such as changes in DNA methylation, histone modification and non-coding RNA expressions, act through regulation of cell-type specific and time-dependent gene expression. Disturbance of such epigenetic marks by environmental stressors may bring about long-term and late-onset health effects, including non-communicable diseases (NCDs). It can further lead to inter-generational effects, such as multigenerational and transgenerational effects, via epigenetic inheritance maintained in the germ cell genome.

This is the bottom line: Doing all the things we suggest in the **BEEMS** protocol, as appropriate to you and your health, can have an impact much later in life on your ability to prevent or mitigate the symptoms of dementia. In effect, you can build muscle memory or molecular memory to call upon when you most need it.

The Molecular Basis of Memory

Brain's Molecular Memory Switch Identified

Further study is needed on the impact of epigenetics for all diseases and disorders. Differences in socio-economic status should also be considered as related to the epigenetic hypothesis of aging-related cognitive levels. Socio-economic factors will hopefully be embraced by researchers, medical practitioners, and funding institutions.

We cannot wait for a vaccine or a pill, nor would we ever support a costly prescription drug, even if it did stop dementia, simply because most people could not afford it. Our approach is more challenging than taking a pill, but it is more affordable and it can be started today.

We believe that through our **BEEMS** approach we have a broader reach as well as a competitive advantage in advancing the state of the epigenetic hypothesis, that is, positioning epigenetics as the fundamental regulator of learning and memory.

The Biology of Belief

Epigenetics – How Does It Work?

Epigenetics: The Science of Change

THE MOST IMPORTANT STUDIES THAT INFORM THE BEEMS PROTOCOL

Medical scientists and practitioners often hesitate to identify the "most important" studies due to limitations of the research methods and populations studied. Nonetheless, we prefer studies with multi-factorial interventions that have been shown to increase cognitive abilities, slow down the progression of mental degradation, and possibly even prevent the onset of dementia.

Two major longitudinal studies provide the context for our approach: The China Study and The Nun Study. These are both critically important studies. The consensus of the two million people who bought the China Study book is that (from the book's jacket cover) "…it is the most influential book ever written on diet and disease."

THE CHINA STUDY

The China Study, conducted in the 1970s by Dr. T. Colin Campbell, has been called the foremost primer of nutrition's impact on health and longevity. Dr. Campbell's interpretation of the research suggests that animal products are the real cause of cancer and other chronic diseases. There are others who disagree with the proposal that all forms of chronic disease can be eliminated by adopting a plant-based diet.

| **The China Study—The Written Report** |
| **Forks Over Knives – The Movie** |

BRAAK'S HYPOTHESIS

Parkinson's disease is strongly linked to the deterioration of the brain's movement center. In 2003, Heiko Braak suggested a new theory of where Parkinson's comes from: the gut! Think of earlier studies, the China Study, and the film *Forks over Knives* while you explore Braak's Hypothesis.

Exploring Braak's Hypothesis of Parkinson's Disease

Disputed Theory on Parkinson's Origin Strengthened

Braak's theory was recently substantiated and reinforced in the article cited earlier on the gut-brain, vagus nerve.

Does Parkinson's Begin in the Gut?

Inflammatory Bowel Disease and inflammation may also be culprits.

Anti–Tumor Necrosis Factor Therapy and Incidence of Parkinson's Disease Among Patients With Inflammatory Bowel Disease

Parkinson's is quickly growing into an epidemic and is believed to be a result of the growth of industrialization around the world.

Are We Facing a Parkinson's Pandemic?

THE NUN STUDY

Professor David Snowdon, the principal investigator of the Nun Study, shows how pathology, plaques, and tangles can be misinterpreted and are not necessarily symptomatic of Alzheimer's Disease. The nuns in this study showed no early symptoms of cognitive decline, and scored normal results on both mental and physical tests.

When the nuns were much younger and initially were entering the convent, they were each asked to write a brief biographical essay. After they died, it was discovered that the essays that were denser, more complex and more fluent were reliable predictors of reduced risk of developing Alzheimer's Disease.

The Nun Study also showed that positive psychology was at work. Positive emotional content expressed in the nuns' essays was strongly associated with longevity.

> **Positive Emotions in Early Life and Longevity:**
> **Findings from the Nun Study**

Two takeaways from this amazing study are 1) develop your "gray matter" (we call this cognitive reserve), and 2) develop and apply positive emotions in all your daily interactions. Being present and mindful is another beneficial learning from the Nun Study.

This study is emblematic of our focus on **BEEMS** as a preventative set of interventions to improve the overall quality of life we can expect. How these nuns lived, ate, exercised, behaved spiritually, demonstrated positive regard for others, and lived in a safe and beautiful environment could all be predictors for mitigation of cognitive decline.

<table>
<tr><td>Nuns Offer Clues to Alzheimer's and Aging</td></tr>
<tr><td>Healthy Aging and Dementia: Findings
from the Nun Study</td></tr>
</table>

PREDIVA STUDY (PREVENTION OF DEMENTIA BY INTENSIVE VASCULAR CARE)

The Dutch PreDIVA study is the first study implementing a multi-domain approach to preventing dementia. However, a popular press headline read, "PreDIVA Trial Falls Short."

This study was initiated in 2009 and was reported by *The Lancet* in 2016. Baffling researchers, there were no reported differences between the group receiving interventions that involved changing smoking habits, diet, exercise, blood pressure, and tailored lifestyle advice; and the control group that received only general medical advice and information. One interpretation of these findings is that people in the Netherlands are generally healthy and have access to high quality care, and thus the population was not ideal for studying.

This study did, however, argue for a research model linking risk factors to dementia, which we see in the FINGER Study, the MAPT Study, and the design of the upcoming POINTER Study. We cover all three studies in the next sections.

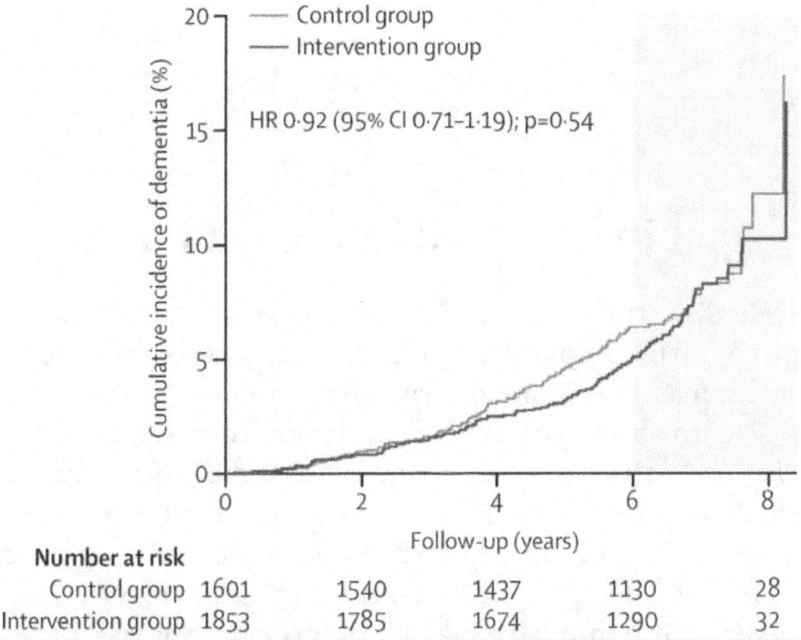

Effectiveness of a 6-year Multidomain Vascular Care Intervention to Prevent Dementia (preDIVA): a Cluster-Randomised Controlled Trial

THE FINGER STUDY

The FINGER Study (Finnish Geriatric Intervention Study to Prevent Cognitive Impairment and Disability) was the first large, long-term and randomized trial with control groups using the multi-factorial approach of preventing dementia through various lifestyle changes and behavioral interventions. This multi-variable approach to preventing dementia used active dietary consultations, exercise regimens, cognitive training, and vascular risk monitoring in a double-blind and randomized trial over two years. It demonstrated that older people at risk of cognitive decline could improve or maintain levels of cognitive functioning later into life than the control group.

This practical approach influenced the U.S. Alzheimer's Association to fund the POINTER Study, which will study the benefits of nutritional counseling, exercise trainers, cognitive training, and social stimulation activities.

All four of these major studies emphasize changing behaviors and lifestyle!

> **The Finnish Geriatric Intervention Study to Prevent Cognitive Impairment and Disability (FINGER): Study Design and Progress**

MAPT RCT (MULTIDOMAIN ALZHEIMER PREVENTIVE TRIAL)

Healthy Aging Through Internet Counseling in The Elderly (HATICE) was used for the French MAPT study. It was a randomized and controlled trial focused on prevention of heart disease and dementia. These two diseases share many risk factors. The multi-domain set of interventions were conducted in three European countries: the Netherlands, France, and Finland.

> **MAPT Study: A Multidomain Approach for Preventing Alzheimer's Disease: Design and Baseline Data**

Nearly 30% of dementia cases start with cardiovascular issues. Risk factors identified were mood, cognitive functioning, and cardiovascular disease. The primary outcomes underscored the importance of improving and monitoring systolic blood pressure, low-density lipoprotein (the "bad" cholesterol which raises risk for heart disease and stroke), and Body Mass Index (BMI). By implementing a multi-domain set of interventions, it was plausible to conclude that the prevalence of dementia and the severity of cognitive decline could be reduced.

This study included heart disease coaching on an interactive internet platform. The interactive interface for participants in this trial helped the study by providing a portal of health for individuals.

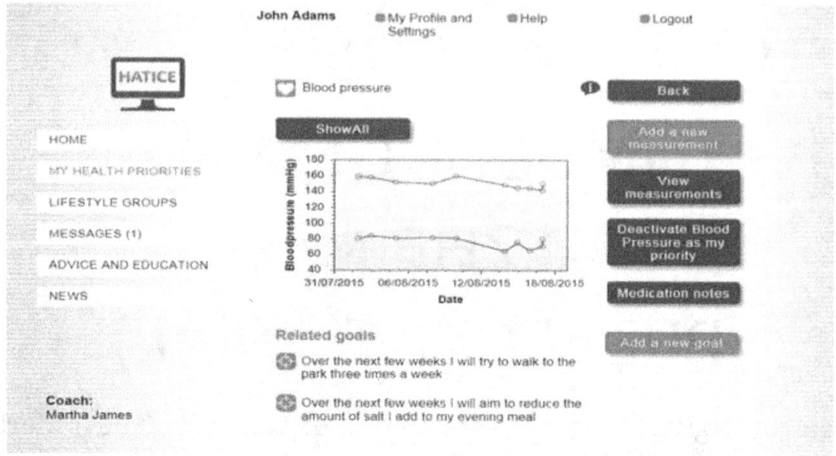

Healthy Ageing Through Internet Counselling in the Elderly: the HATICE Randomised Controlled Trial for the Prevention of Cardiovascular Disease and Cognitive Impairment

Most recently, The Lancet Commission on Dementia Prevention, Intervention, and Care summarized their research:

> In this Commission, we have detailed evidence-based approaches to dementia and its symptoms. Services should be available, scalable, and give value. Professionals and services need to use what works, not use what is ineffective, and be aware of the difference.
>
> Overall, there is good potential for prevention and, once someone develops dementia, for care to be high-quality, accessible, and give value to an underserved, growing population. Effective dementia prevention, intervention, and care could transform the future for society and vastly improve living and dying for individuals with dementia and their

families. Acting now on what we already know can make this difference happen.

(Gill Livingston, Andrew Sommerlad, Vasiliki Orgeta, Sergi G Costafreda, Jonathan Huntley, David Ames, and others "The Lancet," Vol. 390, No. 10113, p.2673–2734 Published: July 19, 2017).

Dementia Prevention, Intervention, and Care

THE POINTER STUDY

Dementia has not been studied uniformly using the gold standard of research design with randomized control groups, all available interventions, and coaching support to change behaviors over time. However, the U. S. Alzheimer's Association in 2018-2019 launched recruiting for the POINTER Study, a $20 million clinical trial designed to test the effects of multiple lifestyle interventions on cognitive decline.

> **U.S. POINTER A Lifestyle Intervention Trial to Support Brain Health and Prevent Cognitive Decline**

The scientific context for this, we believe, involves changing the genotype to a phenotype through behavioral change. In the last two decades, there has been an explosion of scientific evidence supporting this approach.

The Lancet's research parallels the **BEEMS** protocol, as does the Alzheimer's Association's report which summarized modifiable risk factors for cognitive decline and dementia in the *Journal of Alzheimer's and Dementia* (2015). This evidence has encouraged further research into how lifestyle changes might prevent cognitive decline.

> **Bridging the Translation Gap: from Dementia Risk Assessment to Advice on Risk Reduction**

Kaarin J. Anstey, FASSA, is one of Australia's top dementia scientists and is Co-Deputy Director of the ARC Centre of Excellence in Population Ageing Research at the University of New South Wales, Australia, where she is Scientia Professor of Psychology. Dr. Anstey and her colleagues determined and summarized risk assessment values for mid-life and later life subjects and prevention strategies in the *Journal of Prevention Alzheimer's Disease.* She found that a multi-factorial approach to prevention might work in stopping cognitive decline and ultimately, dementia (2015). The following graph is a testament to Dr. Anstey and her colleagues' robust research.

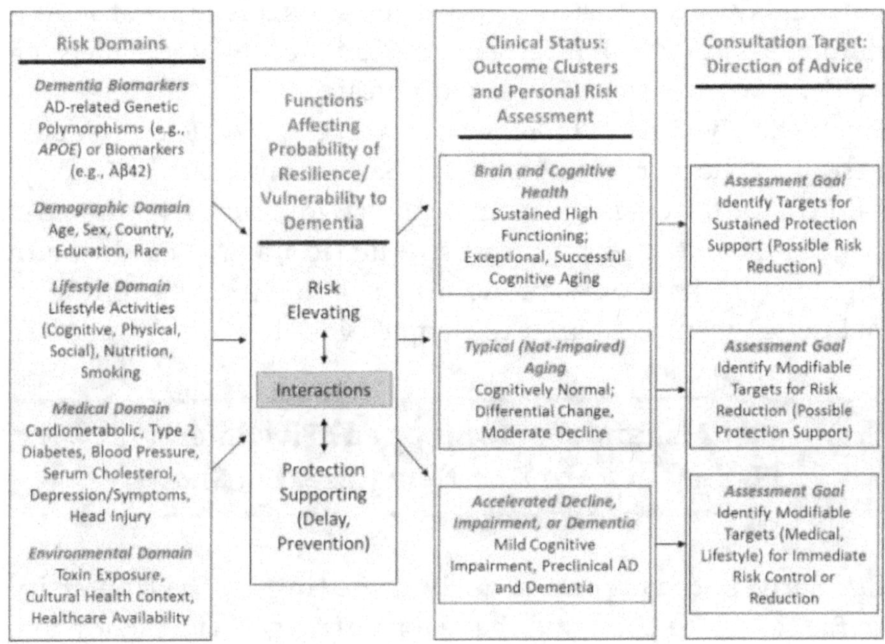

BREAKING NEWS —THIS JUST IN!

On Sunday, July 14, 2019, a press release came out of the Alzheimer's Association International Conference Annual Meeting held in Los Angeles. The headline said, "Can Alzheimer's Be Stopped? Five Lifestyle Behaviors Are Key, New Research Suggests." In short, researchers from Rush University in Chicago said that following life-changing behaviors such as not smoking, regular exercise, cognitive stimulation, and a healthy brain diet results in a 60% reduction in risk of developing Alzheimer's when compared to people who do not follow these lifestyle behaviors.

> **Can Alzheimer's Be Stopped? Five Lifestyle Behaviors Are Key, New Research Shows**

Similarly, a study reported at the same time by the University of Exeter in the UK found that even with a genetic risk for cognitive decline, the incidence of dementia was 32% lower with a healthy lifestyle.

> **Healthy Lifestyle May Offset Genetic Risk of Dementia**

The following study looked at nearly 200,000 subjects over a follow-up period of 8 years. Findings were reported in the prestigious *Journal of the American Medical Association* (JAMA) on

July 14, 2019.

Association of Lifestyle and Genetic Risk with Incidence of Dementia

Finally, a University of California San Francisco study (reported in the same news release) found that smokers could reduce their risk of cognitive decline significantly by quitting.

More Proof that Healthy Lifestyle Reduces Cognitive Impairment, Dementia Risk

According to a press release from the Alzheimer's Association International Conference (AAIC), a combination of healthy habits can lead to increased protection from cognitive decline. "While there is no proven cure or treatment for Alzheimer's, a large body of research now strongly suggests that combining healthy habits promotes good brain health and reduces your risk of cognitive decline," said Maria C. Carrillo, Ph.D., Alzheimer's Association Chief Science Officer.

Additionally, "The research reported today at AAIC gives us attainable, actionable recommendations that can help us all live a healthier life." This book, the **BEEMS** protocol, and our coaching model all provide actionable items that can be initiated today.

Lifestyle Interventions Provide Maximum Memory Benefit When Combined, May Offset Elevated Alzheimer's Risk Due to Genetics, Pollution

The demonstrated value of lifestyle changes reinforces the notion that dementia is a systems-oriented and personal disease. And, just as with heart disease, changing everyday behaviors can result in not only a healthier heart but a healthier mind.

FINAL NOTES

The U.S. POINTER Study is almost identical to what the Epigenesis team proposed over five years ago. After explaining our approach to a fellow researcher, he referred to it as a "kitchen sink" (multi-variable) study. We agreed, saying that changes in a person's complete lifestyle (Body, Emotions, Environment, Mindfulness, and Spirituality) may help in preventing or slowing dementia, and that a multi-factorial approach is the most viable. We are advocating changing behaviors, starting today!

What has been missing from most of these human trials is behavioral coaching through a robust protocol that will reinforce "molecular memory" via epigenetics. Everyone who attempts to change their lifestyle needs help and support. Think of quitting smoking or drinking. Behavioral change is challenging for most people and demands support from all quarters.

As recently as during the last ten years, most medical schools did not teach epigenetics and the role it plays in health and wellness. We think that epigenetics is a true game changer, and just might be a panacea for Alzheimer's in a variety ways.

BEEMS, which is based on epigenetics theory, is inherently a personalized approach to the potential prevention of dementia and mitigating cognitive decline. Personalization is of prime importance, as an approach that works for others may not work for you.

After you complete a lifestyle assessment, speak to your family physician, and make some critical decisions, one of our behavioral health coaches can assist you and support you in developing a personalized plan, and reinforcing the changes you should make to your behavior and environment.

These choices are all up to you.

BEEMS APPROACH
—WHAT YOU
CAN DO NOW!

BEEMS is an innovative health and wellness approach or protocol that incorporates body, emotion, environment, mindfulness, and spirituality into altering this debilitating, costly and progressive disease. Our protocol emerged from the academic literature and these five "buckets" serve as a good framework that encompasses all of the research that we found. The acronym **BEEMS** is an excellent way to remember this protocol. Think of it as a support structure or something you might use to balance yourself when support and balance are needed.

As stated earlier in this eBook, **B** represents the body: exercise, sleep, life-long learning, and nutrition. **E** represents emotion: anger and depression, and modeling "grace under pressure." **E** also represents the environment: the air we breathe, the friends in our world, the place where we live. **M** represents mindfulness: being present, mindful and meditative; and **S** represents our spirituality: a belief in a higher power, God perhaps, or a dedication to the best and highest good of mankind.

We discuss each of these elements in detail in the sections that follow.

Body

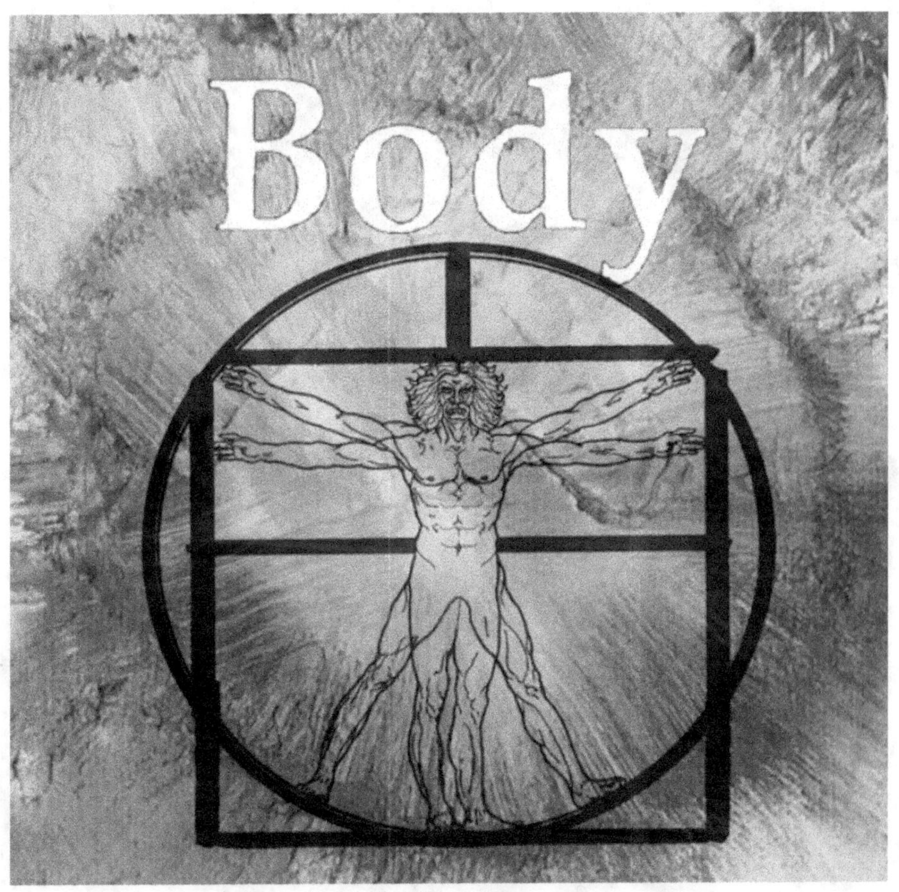

BODY

Research-based evidence on the body is mixed, as different researchers are interested in different aspects that define the "Body." For example, research indicates that there are strong associations between diabetes, Type 2, and dementia. Other researchers study the associations between cardiovascular disease and dementia. And still other researchers look at auto-immune disorders, smoking, obesity, lack of exercise, lack of sex, and their relationships with dementia.

While all these factors should be of concern and should be examined, we ask the question: Do the researchers design the right kinds of studies? Where do sleep, diet, exercise, nutrition, supplements, brain exercises, and a few other promising variables fit into the research design?

Sleep

When we sleep, our body is in a state of rest and our brain may also be in a state of rest, depending on the stage of sleep. Until the invention of electricity, most humans slept long hours at night and their lifestyles revolved around the rising and setting of the sun. They were in tune with the circadian rhythms of the natural world.

In modern society, this is not the case, and the effect on the human body is staggering. A summary of research supports the theory that lack of quality sleep is linked to many health issues. Non-regenerative sleep results in weight gain, irritability, depression, heart disease, strokes, and inflammatory diseases; and perhaps leaves our brains vulnerable to dementia and Alzheimer's disease or other cognitive-neuro disorders.

Sleep is critical to our health and well-being. Think of sleep as the cleaning out of the "trash" we have accumulated during the day.

The relationship between sleep and dementia is being studied quite actively in academic centers around the world. We offer a few good studies below.

Here is the bottom line:

> Larger studies involving more detailed testing are necessary. Medical practitioners need to better understand the complex relationship between sleep and dementia, for example: to understand why people who go on to develop dementia tend to have less REM sleep. REM (rapid eye movement) sleep is a stage of deeper sleep where you are dreaming. Researchers found that if you have less REM sleep, then your chances for developing dementia increase. Finding the underlying cause of these questions could present new avenues by which to diagnose, prevent, or treat dementia, and the only way that this will happen is through continued investment in research.
>
> (Sleep architecture and the risk of incident dementia in the community, Matthew P. Pase, Jayandra J. Himali, Natalie A. Grima, Alexa S. Beiser, Claudia L. Satizabal, Hugo J. Aparicio, Robert J. Thomas, Daniel J. Gottlieb, Sandford H. Auerbach, Sudha Seshadri First published August 23, 2017, "Neurology", DOI: https://doi.org/10.1212/WNL.0000000000004373)

Lack of REM Sleep Linked to an Increased Risk of Dementia

The headlines read that sleep disturbances and loss precede the onset of Alzheimer's disease.

Sleep Disorders Associated With Alzheimer's Disease: A Perspective

We do know that loss of sleep is related to increases in some of the proteins associated with Alzheimer's, e.g., the amyloid-beta and the tau proteins that have been linked to brain damage and an increased risk of Alzheimer's Disease.

Sleep, Alzheimer's Link Explained

But do these proteins cause sleep loss, or does sleep loss cause the buildup of more of these proteins? The direction of the relationship is unclear, but we know there is a relationship or association between the two variables.

In another systematic and meta-analysis of sleep and dementia, the researchers conclude that "Sleep disturbances may predict the risk of incident dementia." This analysis, however, was based upon self-reporting, and so the study needs further validation.

Sleep Disturbances Increase the Risk of Dementia: A Systematic Review and Meta-analysis

Sleep problems are emblematic of Alzheimer's patients but can also lead to other medical problems not associated with dementia or Alzheimer's. Sleep apnea affects overall health and can be challenging. If you snore, talk with your physician. Your physician might have you do a sleep test.

Diet and Nutrition

Eating brain-healthy foods is associated with reduced incidence of Alzheimer's disease. Food is fuel. *High* adherence to any of three diets – MIND, Mediterranean, or DASH – may reduce the risk of Alzheimer's disease. *Moderate* adherence to the MIND diet may also decrease Alzheimer's risk.

There are hundreds if not thousands of websites about diets, new dietary recommendations, anecdotal accounting of foods, and fads. The MIND diet seems to transcend failures of the fleeting promises to lose weight fast. The focus on healthy fats is a key component of the MIND diet and is very relevant in the latest research on dementia. What you read in The China Study also has relevance here: A plant-based diet is good for you.

New MIND Diet May Significantly Protect Against Alzheimer's Disease
What is the MIND Diet?
MIND Diet Associated with Reduced Incidence of Alzheimer's Disease

Other research on diets such as the ketogenic and paleo diets is limited in terms of assessing their value in preventing dementia or slowing its progression. Expect more of these diets to become more mainstream, and our mindset on the value of healthy fat to evolve to include brain health.

Neuroprotective and Disease-Modifying Effects of the Ketogenic Diet

Differences in populations that are under study can affect results. Researchers in Japan found that alterations in dietary patterns may mitigate cognitive decline in an Asian population. This research team found that a higher consumption of soybeans, veggies, and algae, and a lower consumption of rice appear to reduce the risk associated with dementia.

Dietary Patterns and Risk of Dementia

Fiber is also good for you in mitigating causality of disease, as this meta-analysis points out. Although fiber is a well-known health intervention, its effect on brain health is not well-known.

> ## Association Between Dietary Fiber and Lower Risk of All-Cause Mortality: a Meta-Analysis of Cohort Studies
>
> ## Why Is Fiber Good For You?

Eating even healthy foods in large quantities can lead to other problems. The gist of ongoing research unequivocally points to the importance of food moderation and a balanced diet.

> ## In Large Quantities, Health Foods Can Do More Harm than Good

Chronic, heavy alcohol consumption is also associated with Alzheimer's Disease.

> ## Drinking Problems Tied to Higher Risk
>
> ## Largest Study of its Kind Finds Alcohol Use Biggest Risk Factor for Dementia

By contrast, your morning coffee is linked to longevity. Below is a study where the researchers determined that caffeine might be a protective factor in postponing or preventing dementia.

> ## Caffeine as a Protective Factor in Dementia and Alzheimer's Disease

After all that has been reported, be aware that there are limitations with all of these dietary studies.

What we have discovered is that most of the popularly cited studies may not have been conducted long enough, may have too many limitations or too few subjects, may use incorrect measures, and may have confusing outcomes. Fortunately, this has begun to change as concern for the rising rates of dementia increases.

Simply stated, more research needs to be done, and recently the U.S. Congress appropriated more money for dementia studies.

Supplements

Supplements in the forms of oils, pills, powders, and elixirs as additives to our diets are very mainstream now. No longer is a multi-vitamin considered enough. And considering the poor food choices of many people these days, replacing missing micronutrients no longer found in our foods or on our plates might be a field that has great potential for changing brain health and reducing inflammation in all parts of the body.

Some research entirely rejects the notion that daily use of supplements is beneficial.

Study: Multivitamins, Other Common Supplements Have No Health Benefits

This study shows limited evidence for vitamins and improved levels of cognition.

Vitamin and Mineral Supplementation for Preventing Dementia or Delaying Cognitive Decline in People with Mild Cognitive Impairment

Other studies show promise with some supplements such as curcumin and its effect on chronic inflammation.

Efficacy of Curcumin for Age-Associated Cognitive Decline: a Narrative Review of Preclinical and Clinical Studies

---

Some research demonstrates that folic acid can improve levels of cognition and reduces inflammation, a leading indicator of cognitive decline.

The Effects and Potential Mechanisms of Folic Acid on Cognitive Function: a Comprehensive Review

---

Yet, in other studies, there was no impact on levels of cognition with subjects who were already experiencing mild cognitive impairment.

Vitamin and Mineral Supplementation for Preventing Dementia or Delaying Cognitive Decline in People with Mild Cognitive Impairment

---

There are reported research results that show promise for how diet can mitigate levels of cognitive decline with Omega 3. We also looked at levels of Vitamin B and its efficacy in improving levels of cognition. The results seem promising.

B Vitamins and the Brain: Mechanisms, Dose and Efficacy—A Review

Omega 3, etc. Prevents Decline in Gray Matter Volume of the Frontal, Parietal and Cingulate Cortex in Patients with Mild Cognitive Impairment

---

Research evidence is mixed at best. Personal trials with supplements can help you determine what might work for you in visible and measurable areas of your health. These personal benefits might also extend to improved brain health. New research is coming out daily regarding supplements, and book updates will follow the research closely.

Exercise

There have been many studies over the last 20 years evaluating the relationship between physical exercise and the risk of onset of cognitive impairment and dementia, and the impact of exercise on subjects with cognitive impairment or dementia. The outcomes of these studies are not consistent.

Researchers look at a population and examine the relationship between the amount of exercise subjects experience and the proportion of subjects with cognitive impairment in each exercise intensity level at a given point in time. Not surprisingly, more exercise is associated with a lower proportion of subjects with cognitive impairment. The studies mentioned here find a protective association between physical exercise and the onset of cognitive decline.

> **Leisure Time Physical Activity and Dementia Risk: a Dose-Response Meta-Analysis of Prospective Studies**

This study of community dwellers in Canada shows that a high level of physical activity was associated with a reduction of 50% in the incidence of Alzheimer's Disease.

> **Physical Activity and Risk of Cognitive Impairment and Dementia in Elderly Persons**

In the next study, subjects who did not walk daily were 77% more likely to develop dementia than those who walked more than 2 miles every day.

Walking and Dementia in Physically Capable Elderly Men

In Danish women, weekly physical activity reduced risk of cognitive impairment by 23%.

Late-Life Risk Factors for All-Cause Dementia and Differential Dementia Diagnoses in Women: A Prospective Cohort Study

There are several factors that can account for variability in the magnitude of positive effects of exercise, as well as the absence of effects. It is widely accepted that cognitive impairment, often leading to dementia, is influenced by many factors such as cardiovascular status, diabetes, body weight, level of education, diet, and exercise. Exercise is just one of these important factors.

Physical Activity Interventions in Preventing Cognitive Decline and Alzheimer-type Dementia: A Systematic Review

Physical Activity, Cognitive Decline, and Risk of Dementia: 28-year Follow-up of Whitehall II Cohort Study

A healthy lifestyle includes exercise, and it is especially important as we grow older. Several studies suggest that physical exercise may mitigate cognitive decline in those over 50, regardless of their current state of brain health. This meta-analysis of research shows that some types of physical exercise can be considered as alternative therapies.

> **Exercise Interventions for Cognitive Function in Adults Older than 50: a Systematic Review with Meta-Analysis**

Resistance training and mental training seem to improve levels of cognition with subjects who are already experiencing cognitive decline.

> **The Study of Mental and Resistance Training (SMART) Study—Resistance Training and/or Cognitive Training in Mild Cognitive Impairment: a Randomized, Double-Blind, Double-Sham Controlled Trial**

Nearly every major study underscores the value of some form of exercise, even if it is just walking for 10 minutes a day. Whether it is a fast-paced cardio workout, lifting weights, or doing resistance training, almost any form of exercise is a good thing.

The next section of this book reminds us of the need to be very careful when engaged in exercise. Many individuals have experienced serious head injuries. Traumatic Brain Injuries (TBIs) and concussions are the most common injuries that individuals may face in life.

Traumatic Brain Injury and Dementia

Traumatic Brain Injury (TBI) affects nearly 2% of the U.S. population, and it costs our nation billions of dollars. It has been said that TBI might be the oldest form of disorder known to mankind. Ever since David and Goliath, we have seen the deleterious and invasive results of concussions. And, sadly, today there is no standard of care for those most impacted by this. Our children and our seniors suffer the most. Be it a bump, a fall, a blow (a rock or punch to the head), a jolt, or a sports injury, all can trigger life-long disabilities.

Traumatic Brain Injury & Concussion

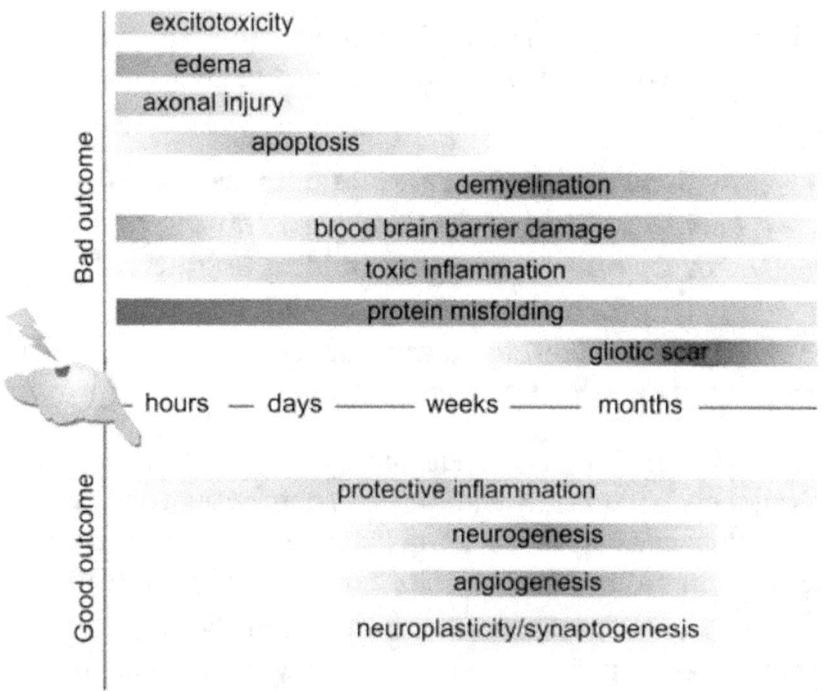

Chronic Impact of Traumatic Brain Injury on Outcome and Quality of Life: a Narrative Review

The Centers for Disease Control recently published a book that delves deeper into this tragic injury, but sadly does not proffer any solid, evidence-based treatments. Future studies will be offered here as they become available. We applaud Congress and the CDC for bringing this terrible disorder into the public conversation. We must do more about TBI for our veterans, children, and seniors. TBI is something that might change their lives, and also might trigger the comorbidities that often accompany TBI.

Traumatic Brain Injury In the US: Emergency Department Visits, Hospitalizations and Deaths 2002–2006

In the publication, *Journal of American Physicians and Surgeons*, Volume 22, Number 2, Summer 2017, the authors argue for the efficacy of Hyperbaric Oxygen Therapy (HBOT). They say, "Many recent reports provide evidence for its effectiveness in promoting repair of neurologic injuries, whether traumatic or anoxic." The authors draw from many good studies, and HBOT is not just a therapy for TBI, but is beneficial in treating several other disorders or physical problems as well.

The Next Generation in Brain Recovery and Neuroregeneration

Hyperbaric oxygen therapy is not without its controversies; however, for one of our authors, HBOT has been key in treating the aftereffects of TBI. After 90 sessions, there has been a marked increase in his ability to speak, reason, focus, and live without concomitant side effects or comorbidities.

What Is Hyperbaric Oxygen Therapy Good for?

The journal *Neurology* helps us better understand the implications of HBOT and the general findings of several clinical trials. The authors conclude that:

> Hyperbaric oxygen and hyperbaric air have demonstrated therapeutic effects on mTBI/PPCS (Persistent Post Concussion Symptoms) and can alleviate posttraumatic stress dis-

order symptoms secondary to a brain injury in 5 out of 5 peer-reviewed clinical trials. The current use of pressurized air (1.2–1.3 ATA) as a placebo or sham in clinical trials biases the results due to biological activity that favors healing.

You will recall that earlier we said TBI could lead to dementia. Here is what a federally sponsored research study concludes:

Traumatic brain injury (TBI) is among the earliest illnesses (dating back nearly 3 million years) described in human history and remains a major source of morbidity and mortality in the modern era. It is estimated that 2% of the US population lives with long-term disabilities due to a prior TBI, and incidence and prevalence rates are even higher in developing countries. One of the most feared long-term consequences of TBIs is dementia, as multiple epidemiologic studies show that experiencing a TBI in early or mid-life is associated with an increased risk of dementia in late life. The best data indicate that moderate and severe TBIs increased risk of dementia between '2 and 4-fold.'

Dementia resulting from Traumatic Brain Injury. What Is the Pathology?

Even mild TBI might raise one's risk for dementia (may almost double the risk) as reported in the *JAMA Neurology Journal* in May 2018.

Even Mild TBI Might Raise Dementia Risk
Association of Mild Traumatic Brain Injury with and Without Loss of Consciousness With Dementia in US Military Veterans

TBI is not something to be trifled with. Symptoms may not

show up for months, and getting help quickly is very important. TBI is the most well-established environmental risk factor for dementia. Head injury is also a risk factor for Alzheimer's Disease. Hospitals need to start including TBI information in discharge orders, e.g., what to be aware of and what to be watchful for after a patient has left carrying all their X-rays to their neurologist! What may happen over time could easily be avoided with advance notice, education and preparation.

> **Head Injury as a Risk Factor for Alzheimer's Disease: The Evidence 10 Years on, a Partial Replication**
>
> **Head Injury as a Risk Factor for Dementia and Alzheimer's Disease: A Systematic Review and Meta-Analysis of 32 Observational Studies**

From the research conclusions:

> Head injury is a risk factor for AD. The magnitude of the risk is proportional to severity and heightened among first-degree relatives of AD patients. The influence of head injury on the risk of AD appears to be greater among persons lacking APOE-epsilon4 compared with those having one or two epsilon4 alleles, suggesting that these risk factors may have a common biologic underpinning.

Do not let a concussion go by without examination by your primary care physician and/or a neurologist. You might not feel any symptoms for months. Be sure to keep watch over the longer term for changes in mood or behavior, or other symptoms of TBI.

We have come a long way since that first caveman struck his fellow human in the head with a club. But a slip on the ice and hitting your head is so much more than just a fall. For more information on falls and especially fall prevention, please look at this, and this...

> ## National Falls Prevention Resource Center

> ## Evidence-Based Falls Prevention Programs

Even losing a tooth can be considered a risk factor for dementia. Inflammation was pointed out earlier as a risk factor. What is closest to the brain? Your mouth and your ears. And what can become infected readily with the result being inflammation? A tooth infection can be something you can easily avoid.

> ## Tooth Loss as a Risk Factor for Dementia: Systematic Review and Meta-analysis of 21 Observational Studies

We finish our discussion of TBI with a story, accessible here with permission and with invaluable input from one parent's experience with his son's TBI. There is no doubt that anyone who has suffered from a concussion, be it the result of a car accident, a fall down stairs, or being thrown from a horse, is being attended to more rigorously – possibly more rigorously now than ever before.

We wanted to bring attention to traumatic brain injury because anyone can hit their head during almost any activity, and most people, we have discovered, do not know what the symptoms of a TBI are or how best to manage it. It is a life-changing event, as we know from personal experience.

> ## Fighting the "TBI Wars": New Alternatives for TBI Survivors

Cognitive Therapies and Exercise for Your Brain

Exercising the brain shows some promise and is the subject of several research studies. However, other studies do not agree, especially when the studies involve people already showing signs of mild cognitive impairment. The authors here conclude that "Currently available evidence does not allow us to determine whether or not computerized cognitive training will prevent clinical dementia or improve or maintain cognitive function in those who already have evidence of cognitive impairment."

> ## Computerized Cognitive Training for Preventing Dementia in People with Mild Cognitive Impairment

The authors cite several methodological problems with most of the research, even though some individual studies demonstrated high levels of impact.

> ## Does Scientific Evidence Show Brain Training Works?

Brain games and brain training methods are proliferating, but until recently there was not much evidence as to which methodologies work and which ones do not. We did find one review in the literature that met our "gold standard" for research rigor. Posit Science training was found to improve processing speed, memory, and reasoning in the brain in significant and positive ways.

> ## Enhancing Cognitive Functioning in Healthy Older Adults: a Systematic Review of the Clinical Significance of Commercially Available Computerized Cognitive Training in Preventing Cognitive Decline

Another review sheds light on the differences between Posit Science and other brain training games.

> ## This Is the Only Type Of Brain Training

That Works, According To Science

Still other researchers found equivocal results for any brain training program.

Do "Brain-Training" Programs Work?

The Weak Evidence Behind Brain-Training Games

Our conclusion is that, while brain training may not work for everyone, each day can become a day that offers a wide variety of activities, including exercise and inquiry. You may discover something that makes you stronger and healthier, even if the science is lacking.

THIS JUST IN !

Brain State Technologies (https://cereset.com/) and it's Founder/CEO, Lee Gerdes, have invented a radical new approach to healing brain injuries through sound waves. Our lead author, Barry Spiker can attest to its efficacy. You may want to go their website and read some of the important research papers such as https://clinicaltrials.gov/ct2/show/NCT03649958.

Several states in the US have a Brain Injury Alliance (https://www.usbia.org). Plus there is another national organization the Brain Injury Association of America (https://biausa.org). Brain injuries, though the most common reason for entering an emergency room, are some of the most misunderstood, misdiagnosed and most poorly financed and researched injuries anywhere in the world.

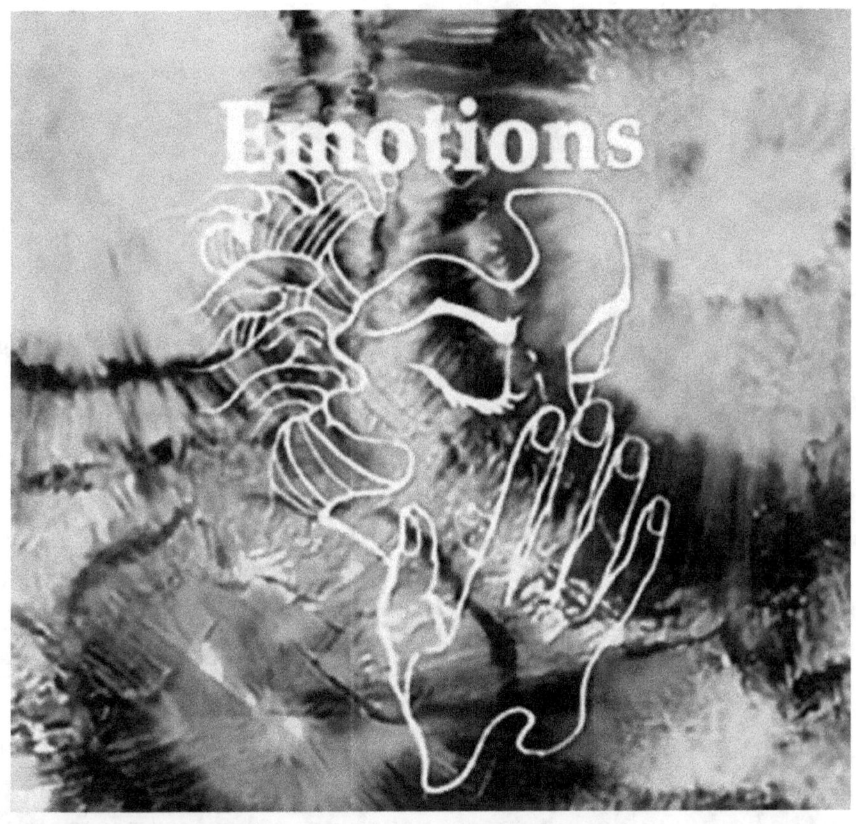
Emotions

EMOTIONS

Emotions are difficult to address with some people. Our emotions are reactions in our brains and bodies to thoughts and stimuli in our environment. The scientific community and many people are just beginning to understand how emotions create stress and how stress can impact an individual's health and well-being. How an individual handles or responds to their emotions can increase or reduce stress and anger, as well as elation and joy. These responses can impact a person's entire life.

Understanding stress and emotional reactions is extremely important! Researchers look at oxidative stress specifically to better understand the effects of stress on the body's immune functions. Oxidation is normal and necessary and takes place in the body. Oxidative stress occurs when there is an imbalance between free radical activity and antioxidant activity. When functioning properly, free radicals help fight off pathogens. Pathogens lead to infections and can do damage to DNA and proteins in the body. Proteins, lipids, and DNA make up a large part of the body such that over time, damage to these elements can lead to a vast number of diseases. Diseases such as heart disease, cancer, diabetes, high blood pressure, Parkinson's, and Alzheimer's are all potential consequences of higher than normal levels of stress.

Emotional Intelligence--EQ

We start this section with Emotional Intelligence (EQ) because the essence of EQ is defined as how one chooses to manage their emotions in response to stimuli in their environment. The environment itself also influences an individual's response to and the impact of stress.

Emotional Intelligence is about being aware of, managing, and expressing emotions effectively in relationships. Like other forms of intelligence, emotional intelligence can have a significant, beneficial impact on mitigating cognitive decline. Learning to navigate and manage emotions is useful for reducing stress, increasing empathy, developing resilience, building an ability to increase positive emotions, becoming more present and mindful, and developing problem-solving abilities that can enhance life. Using EQ in these ways can significantly influence how well a person regulates stress, anger, depression, frustration, and anxiety.

Assessing your Emotional Intelligence can be as simple as evaluating your reaction when someone says something that you strongly disagree with. A person could react negatively and escalate the conversation into an argument, or could respond thoughtfully and take responsibility for the response. Here are a few questions you might want to ask yourself to better manage your EQ.

Do you listen well? Do you think before you respond? Are you caring, compassionate, and considerate? Do you attend to your inner guidance and react in your own best interest? Do you make good decisions while considering the current and unintended consequences of those decisions? Do people describe you as happy and optimistic, compassionate and empathetic? Are you prepared to manage your emotions in the event of the worst possible outcomes? Do you keep your cool and stay calm when dealing with stressful situations?

What Is Emotional Intelligence?

Emotional Intelligence Scales

How Emotionally Intelligent Are You?

Test your Emotional Intelligence with our Free EQ Quiz

If you understand your emotions, you can better regulate them. The following two web sites underscore the notion that developing EQ is fast becoming a movement in personal and professional arenas.

Six Seconds EQ Network

Elementally EQ

For those who have a diagnosis of dementia (as well as their caretakers), there is good advice in the following resource on how best to manage emotions and cope with others' anger, frustration, and depression.

Dementia Care Central

Stress, Anger, and Depression

We know that stress, anger, and depression are associated with dementia. Research shows that these attitudes and situations can be reversed.

Chronic Stress Could Lead to Depression and Dementia, Scientists Warn

Stress Might Be Just as Unhealthy as Junk Food to Digestive System

Anger, depression, frustration, anxiety, and stress can be observable behavioral signs that emerge in a person showing early indications of mild cognitive decline or early signs of dementia. If you see these behaviors escalating in yourself or your loved ones, it is worth addressing. All these emotions are on display by individuals and family members when a person receives the devastating diagnosis of Alzheimer's or other dementia. Depression is also a risk factor for dementia; that is, if an individual has suffered from depression, there appears to be a greater risk of developing dementia.

Stress, Meditation, and Alzheimer's Disease Prevention: Where The Evidence Stands
Is Your Stress Changing my Brain? Stress Isn't Just Contagious; It Alters the Brain on a Cellular Level

As we age, there also may be differences in how moods and emotions change for men versus women. The relationship between depression and dementia or Alzheimer's disease tends to be stronger for men as they get older; however, it is unclear whether depression becomes more prominent when someone is suffering from dementia.

Very often, we fail to pay attention to our feelings. A first step in understanding whether feelings and behaviors are related to dementia is to recognize them. If individuals and those around them recognize changes in emotion, then the possible reasons for mood disturbance can be narrowed. But how do we begin to recognize changes in mood or emotions when confronted by the potential for serious health concerns?

Fortunately, there are straightforward diagnostic tools for anger, anxiety, and depression that take only a few minutes. The Duke University Anxiety-Depression scale (DUKE-AD) is an easily self-administered diagnostic (you can take it quickly, and the scaling result can recognize and verify anxiety and depression).

Duke Anxiety-Depression Scale (DUKE-AD)

Similarly, there are tests or surveys that can help determine if someone is suffering from unfocused and clinical levels of anger.

The Clinical Anger Scale (CAS) is an objective, valid, self-reporting instrument that measures the psychological symptoms relevant in the understanding and treatment of clinical anger.

Clinical Anger Scale (CAS)

The following symptoms of anger are measured by the CAS: anger now, anger about the future, anger about failure, anger about things, angry-hostile feelings, anger about self, anger misery, wanting to hurt others, shouting at people, annoying others, irritation, social interference, decision interference, alienating others, work interference, sleep interference, fatigue, appetite interference, health interference, thinking interference, and sexual interference.

Beck Depression Inventory

Even uncontrollable laughter can be a sign of some form of a cognitive challenge that shows up as a change in our behavior.

(Overview: Assess Depression Age Range: 13 through 80 years Administration: 5 minutes; self-administered, or verbally by a trained administrator Scoring Options: Manual scoring or Q-global Scoring & Reporting Publication Date: 1996.)

Beck Depression Inventory

Understanding Uncontrollable Crying or Laughing

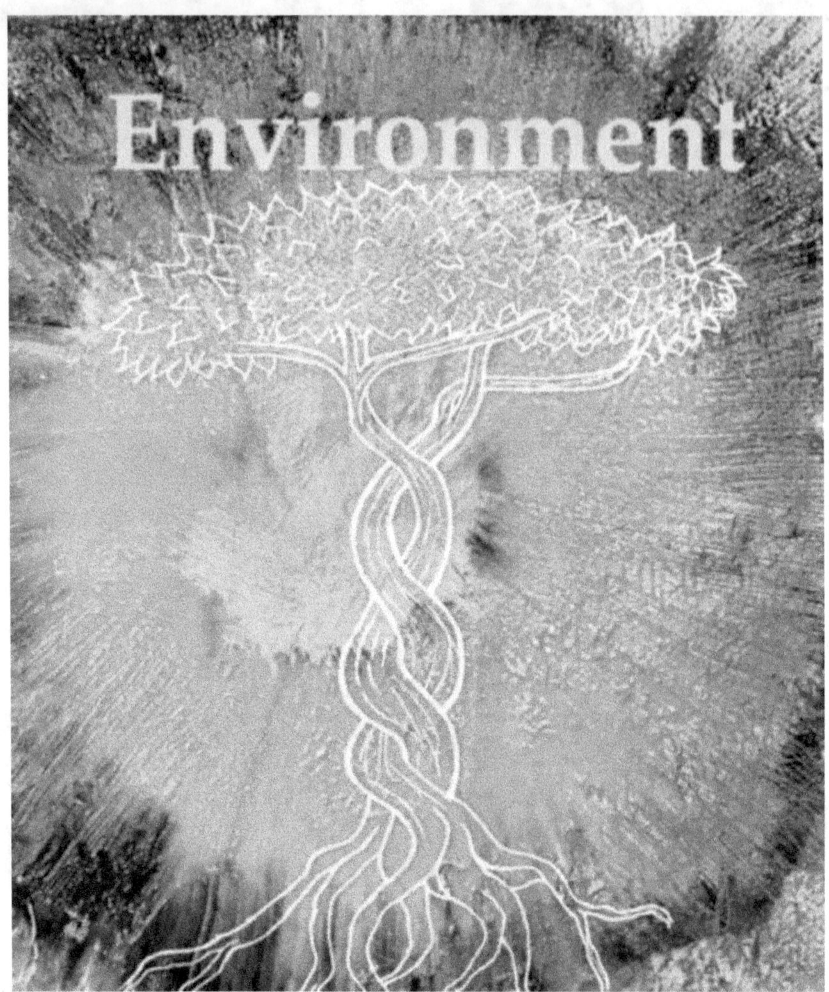
Environment

ENVIRONMENT

Environmental factors may affect the onset and progression of Alzheimer's disease, other dementias, and cognitive decline. This may simply be a consequence of the geographic region that is part of the world you live in and attributes of the people around you. The question is, does the place you live matter when you attempt to improve your health and mitigate cognitive decline and different types of dementia? The likely answer is yes, but whether this is the right answer for you may also depend on specific aspects of health that are of concern.

Most researchers have included single environmental stressors when investigating these issues, and some results show that combined multiple environmental health stressors have a greater impact on health than single stressors. A research group has proposed a tool, Combined Environmental Stressors' Exposure (CENSE), to assess combined exposure to environmental health stressors in urban areas.

> **CENSE: A tool to Assess Combined Exposure to Environmental Health Stressors in Urban Areas**

CENSE addresses co-exposures in a holistic way for urbanites and considers a person's activities and relative exposure to or intake of environmental stressors.

CENSE communicates co-exposure in a trackable manner for urban microenvironments. The outcomes from using the CENSE tool are demonstrated in an example from Thessaloniki, Greece. The results (insights and outcomes) of this test case are validated by the fact that both health stressors and local characteristics were evaluated in the test case. These results could have broader implications due to the holistic approach taken. The goal was to address combined outcomes from 1) exposure to multiple health stressors and 2) control of an environment with those same stressors.

> ## How Our Surroundings Can Help or Hinder Active Lifestyles

In 2017, *The Guardian* printed the headline: "Living Near Heavy Traffic Increases Dementia Risk." CENSE is presented. The tool bridges the gap between chemical and physical health stressors.

> ## Living Near Heavy Traffic Increases Risk of Dementia

Researchers "found that those who live closest to major traffic arteries were up to 12% more likely to be diagnosed with dementia – a small but significant increase in risk." We know that living near highway traffic can increase your exposure to smog and air pollution, noise pollution, and can increase a general awareness of multiple stimuli in the immediate environment.

> ## Living Near Major Roads and the Incidence of Dementia, Parkinson's Disease, and Multiple Sclerosis: a Population-Based Cohort Study

> ## Leading Causes of Death in Nonmetropolitan and Metropolitan Areas— United States, 1999–2014

Neighborhood environments, mobility, light, noise, smells, your own personal space, and the people around you all contribute to or detract from health and wellness. We all know of places where the toxicity levels are so high that no one can live there. Chernobyl and the Love Canal have both been impacted by toxic levels of chemicals or worse.

Neighborhood Environments, Mobility, and Health: Towards a New Generation of Studies in Environmental Health Research

The Economic Innovation Group (EIG) has demonstrated that the states of Alabama, Arkansas, Louisiana, Mississippi, and West Virginia are the most economically distressed states in the US.

Economic Innovation Group

EIG reports that people living in "prosperous" zip codes tend to have social resources that those in "distressed" zip codes do not have. These resources include "access to fresh and nutritious foods, cleaner air, and high-quality schools."

From their analysis, EIG found that those living in prosperous counties have lifespans that are an average of 5 years longer than those living in economically distressed areas. Because people in economically distressed areas have fewer resources, EIG attributed the shorter lifespan to lower quality of life and healthcare.

This conclusion presents a dilemma: Living in a rural environment may basically be healthier, but a city environment offers more amenities and better access to quality healthcare.

Hospital Environments

Access to health care is a crucial consideration for people, especially when they are older and may need to be close to medical professionals and emergency care.

Hospitals are located predominantly in urban areas. Rural areas tend have fewer services available. The geographic location of a hospital usually determines its size, services, demographics, employees, and other factors that contribute to quality of care. Urban hospitals, which represent 62% of all hospitals, serve in densely populated areas, often with several competitors nearby. These hospitals vary in size from under 100 beds to over 500 beds. Rural hospitals are smaller (100 or fewer beds); they have smaller budgets and fewer personnel.

Rural hospitals tend to serve more Medicare, Medicaid, and uninsured patients. They are more likely to be designated Critical Access Hospitals by the Centers for Medicare and Medicaid Services (CMS). Critical Access Hospitals make up about 72% of all regional hospitals. These hospitals have fewer than 25 beds and are typically located at least 35 miles from the next hospital. Both urban and rural hospitals may be designated Safety-Net Hospitals by CMS based on the proportion of charity care provided. As of 2017, these hospitals receive extra funds from CMS to help cover their operating costs.

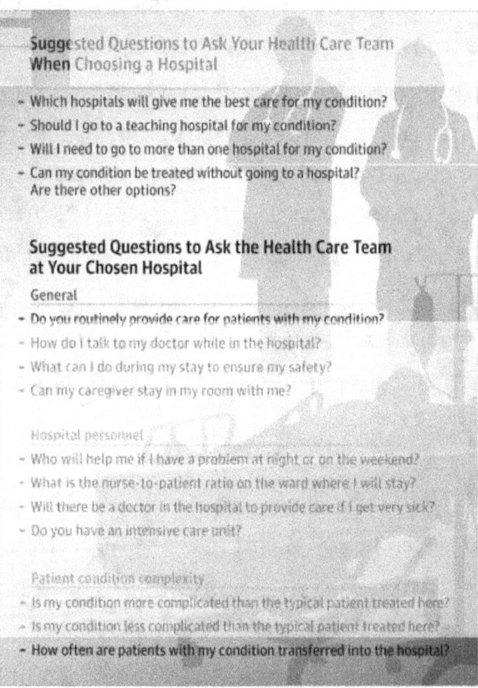

Types of Hospitals in the US

BARRY K SPIKER PHD

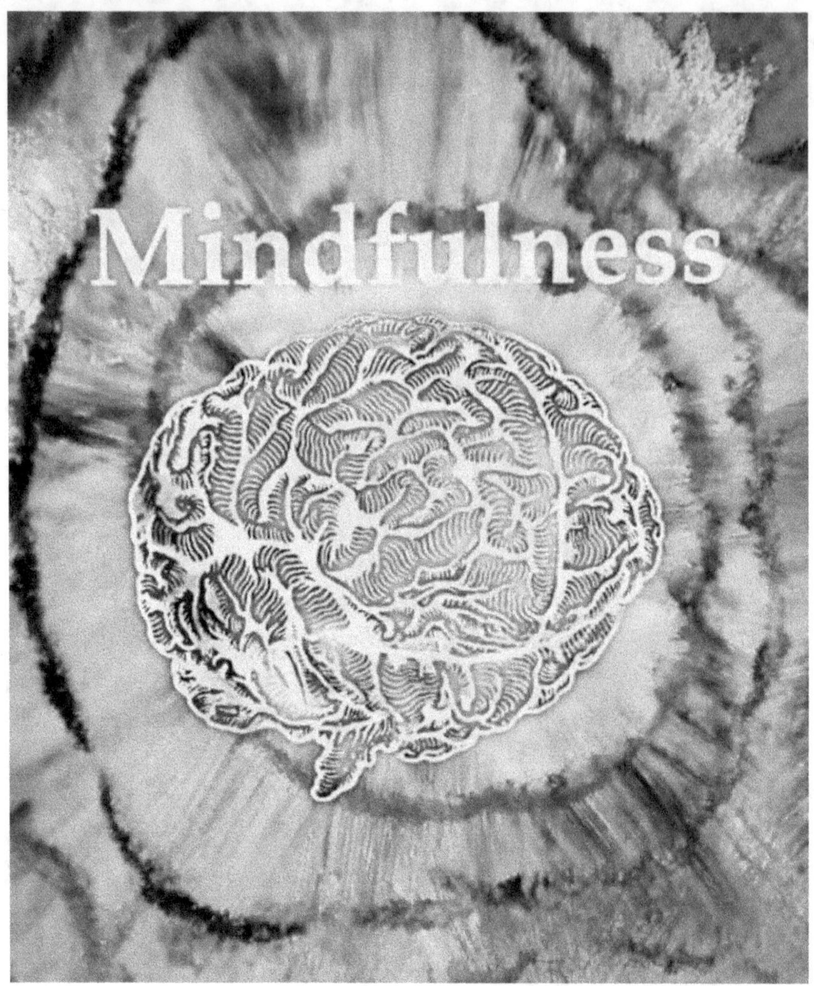

MINDFULNESS

Mindfulness means paying attention to the present. Some research suggests that the practice of mindfulness and mindful meditation mitigates stress, anger, and self-destructive behaviors. Mindfulness focuses people on the present, foments pleasure, and induces relaxation.

If you happen to own a dog, you can readily get an idea of what mindfulness is the next time you lock eyes with your dog. Your dog is not distracted; it is focused entirely on you!

> ## Mindfulness and Being in the Moment

Mindfulness is seen as another word for meditation. Preliminary evidence suggests that meditation can offset age-related cognitive decline and improves the quality of one's life.

> ## What is Mindfulness? A Psychologist Explains

Although results are mixed, the practice of mindfulness has been shown to have health benefits. Whether or not mindfulness affects the progression or severity of Alzheimer's disease, the practice of mindfulness will not harm you.

If you happen to own a dog, you can readily get an idea of what mindfulness is the next time you lock eyes with your dog. Your dog is not distracted; it is focused on you!

> ## Look after Your Mental Health Using Mindfulness

In the United Kingdom, public health stakeholders and health-care givers recommend mindfulness as a part of the National Institute for Health and Care Excellence (NICE) Clinical Guidelines. This very simple questionnaire can enlighten you further.

> ## Mindfulness: It can be Easy to Rush Through Life without Stopping to Notice Much

This short video is a resource that will help you better understand what is needed in order to begin practicing mindfulness.

> ## The Science Behind Mindfulness Meditation

Another video is a brief introduction to meditation as a "superpower." This video will lead you to several guided meditations that you can begin to do right now.

> ## Why Mindfulness Is a Superpower: An Animation

> ## Happify is the Single Destination for Effective, Evidence-based Solutions for Better Emotional Health and Wellbeing in the 21st Century

The Diagnostics of Mindfulness

Freely available diagnostics vary in their emphasis (bias), and have limitations in their methodologies. Nonetheless, it can be very useful to take tests to compare results even if they are not scientifically rigorous. (Note that some websites require you to register to access their content.)

> ## Personality Assessment in the Diagnostic Manuals: On Mindfulness, Multiple Methods,

and Test Score Discontinuities

Potential Benefits of Mindfulness-based Interventions in Mild Cognitive Impairment and Alzheimer's Disease: an Interdisciplinary Perspective

The previous two articles are simply summaries and require that you purchase the article in order to read it in its entirety.

We know that stress, anxiety, and depression are potential markers for dementia. Research indicates that stress, anxiety, and depression can be reversed. Mindfulness is one way to reverse those feelings.

Following is a beginner's guide to meditation. It is a bit of a cartoon and begins with learning how to breathe.

Meditation 101: A Beginner's Guide

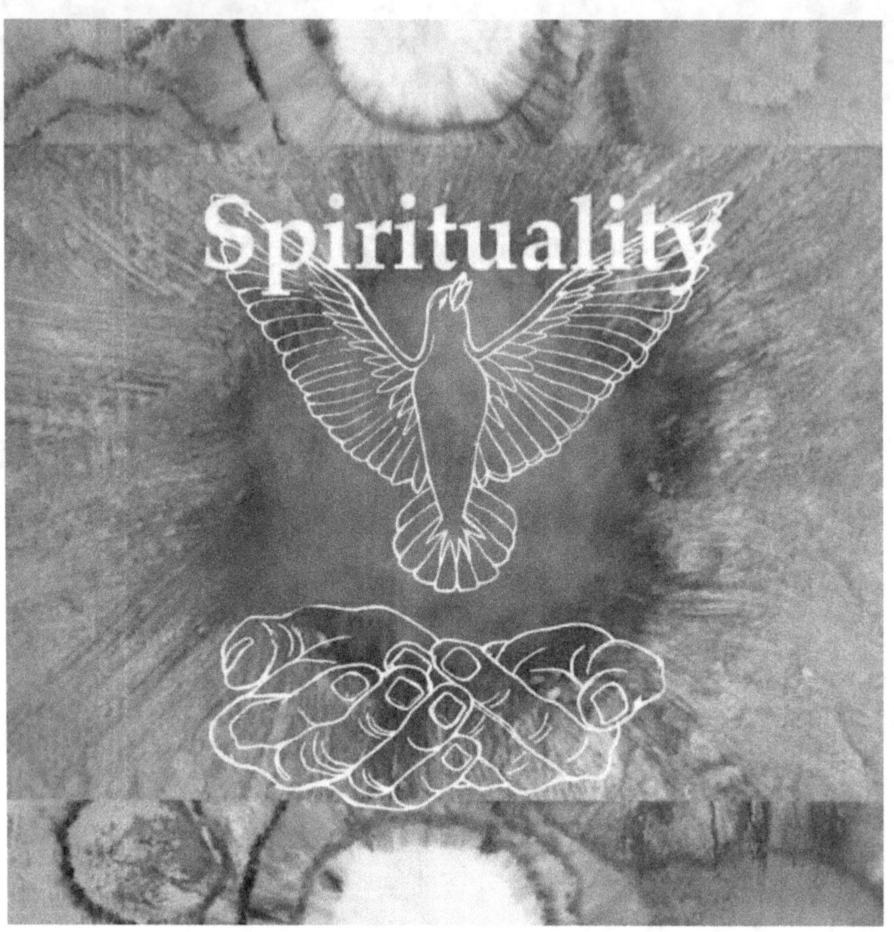
Spirituality

SPIRITUALITY

Spirituality and Dementia

It was in the Fall of 1998 and my friend Judi Neal and I were chatting about upcoming professional meetings where we might meet. Judi was a colleague of mine at Honeywell and had gone on to lead the Walton Institute of Spirituality in Business in Arkansas. But I am getting ahead of myself.

In November, I had met Judi and several other luminaries in

Puerta Vallarta for the 3rd International Conference on Business and Consciousness. We had just sat down to lunch when Deepak Chopra joined us.

A lively discussion ensued and soon "spirituality" was on the tongues of nearly 400 business and spiritual leaders for the next five days. It was Barry's introduction to spirit in the workplace and became the foundation of his work in organizational development. It is now the anchor to the **BEEMS** protocol which is a systemic view of healing and a prophylaxis for mitigating dementia.

Deepak discussed spirituality and the current Covid 19 virus, which is akin to what we might suggest when a family member is diagnosed with a form of dementia https://www.cnbc.com/2020/04/03/deepak-chopra-the-coronavirus-and-need-for-spiritual-wellness.html. As he says, do not give into fear and panic when presented with a possible life-changing event.

We operationalize or define spirituality as something you look to for comfort and something greater than yourself. Whether it be a form of religion or a belief in a higher power, the research literature is large and growing. Beuscher and Beck did a comprehensive literature review of spirituality in coping with early-stage Alzheimer's disease and reported their research in the "Journal of Clinical Nursing" in 2008 Volume 17, Issue 5a, (/doi/10.1111/jcn.2008.17.issue5a/ issuetoc) pages 88–97, March 2008. The authors assert that maintaining a sense of normalcy and preserving self worth are effective coping strategies for a person with Alzheimer's. We could not agree more.

Spirituality and the mindfulness research merge at this point and there is a great deal of evidence suggesting that spirituality is associated with faster healing, easier coping and greater understanding of both patient and caregiver. In fact, higher levels of religiosity seem to correlate with a slower rate of cognitive and behavioral decline for the patient and caregiver https://doi.org/10.2174/156720510791383886.

Emotional/Psychological/Spiritual Instruments

From the abstract:

> The Body-Mind-Spirit Well-Being Inventory (BMSWBI)... comprises four scales: physical distress, daily functioning, affect, and spirituality... Factor analysis indicates that (a) positive and negative affect form two distinct factors; and (b) spirituality comprises three different aspects, tranquility, resistance to disorientation, and resilience. Spirituality is positively associated with mental well-being, positive affect, satisfaction with life, and hope; but negatively associated with negative affect and perceived stress. These results suggest that the inventory may be used to assess different dimensions of health satisfactorily.

> ### The Measurement of Body-Mind-Spirit Well-Being, Social Work in Healthcare

FACIT is a non-profit organization focused primarily on cancer. FACIT means Functional Assessment of Cancer Therapy. There may be be additional instruments represented here that are useful for any chronic illness. We particularly like the FACIT subscale for spiritual well-being.

FACIT Spiritual Wellbeing Sub-Scale

ALTERNATIVE THERAPIES AND DEMENTIA

In this section, we explore some alternative therapies. Art, animal assistance, dance, light, music, and medical cannabis have been shown to slow dementia or mitigate cognitive decline, and assist with the effects or symptoms of dementia. These therapies are not well understood, they are controversial, and studies inherently have poor applications of methodology and limitations in research design.

Alternative therapies need to be researched and studied by scientists and experts. There are currently largely "one-shot" case studies which are observational studies. All science starts with an observation and hypotheses to test, so it is not a bad place to start.

We recommend that you always speak candidly with your doctor, do your own research online, and speak to others who have experience with the therapy that you want to try. If your doctor does not know about the therapy, then they will likely be able to refer you to a colleague who can be helpful. The statistics (and science) often used in published research can be daunting. Ask someone for help.

Also, it is always best to be discerning. For example, research published in the journal *Clinical Nursing Research* on February 14, 2018, on animal-assisted interventions and dementia is included below. One-day rental cost from the publisher is $40.00

for the article. If you do not rent the article to find out what is in it, you cannot determine if what the abstract claims is based on good research, or if instruments that were both valid and reliable were used in the research. One would think results are indeed what the abstract claims, but this is not necessarily the case. It is always best to be discerning.

Art Therapy

Conducting a study in art therapy as a modality or intervention to slow cognitive decline is unfortunately rife with individualism and non-reliable approaches. There are very few randomized controlled trials, and most of the studies are qualitative as opposed to quantitative. There is little research that demonstrates the efficacy of art in aiding dementia patients. Most studies are case-based, but there are a few that show promise.

> **Outcome Studies on the Efficacy of Art Therapy: A Review of Findings**

For people who already have dementia, art therapy is a welcome intervention. The therapeutic aspects of art seem to impact different areas of the brain than areas where dementia resides.

> **Art Therapy and Neuroscience Blend: Working with Patients Who Have Dementia**

In this short film, we see the amazing impact that creating art can have on someone working through the various stages of dementia.

> **Painting in Twilight: An Artist's Escape from Alzheimer's**

The Alzheimer's Association of Orange County (California) has created a way for Alzheimer's patients to express themselves differently than using language. This is a therapy for those already experiencing some form of cognitive decline.

Memories in the Making: Using art as a Communication Tool for People with Memory Loss

While licensed therapists should lead Art Therapy, just coloring with crayons can be fulfilling as well.

Animal Assisted Therapy (AAT)

The following research on animal-assisted therapy (AAT) and dementia was published in the journal, *Clinical Nursing Research*, on February 14, 2018.

Quoting directly from the abstract:

> This review discusses the relationship between animal-assisted interventions (AAI) and behavioral and psychological symptoms of dementia (BPSD). A systematic search was conducted within CINAHL, Web of Science CAB Abstracts, PubMed, Abstracts in Social Gerontology, Google Scholar, and PsycINFO for primary research articles. A total of 32 studies were included in the final review. Variation was noted in study designs and in study setting. 27 of 32 studies used dogs as the intervention. Agitation/aggression showed a significant decrease in 9 of 15 studies. 11 of 12 studies demonstrated increased social interaction with AAI. Mood had mixed results in nine studies. Quality of life was increased in three of four studies. Resident activity and nutritional intake were each increased in two studies. Animal-assisted activities/interventions showed a strong positive effect on social behaviors, physical activity, and

dietary intake in dementia patients and a positive effect on agitation/aggression and quality of life.

(Clinical Nursing Research, 2019 Jan;28(1):9-29. doi: 10.1177/1054773818756987. Epub 2018 Feb 14. Animal-Assisted Intervention and Dementia: A Systematic Review. Yakimicki ML1, Edwards NE1, Richards E1, Beck AM1)

The bottom line is that animals are good to have around, especially if you are concerned with agitation, aggression, moodiness, social interaction or quality of life.

Animal-Assisted Intervention and Dementia: A Systematic Review

In a meta-analysis (49 out of 250 published studies) published in a refereed journal, it was found that AAT can have a positive effect on several disorders ranging from autism to struggles with emotional well-being. Positive outcomes demonstrated moderate-sized effects, and it was found that AAT might be combined with other non-pharmacological studies to increase the effectiveness of this intervention. Animal-assisted therapy has a long history.

Animal-Assisted Therapy: A Meta-Analysis

In the *American Journal of Geriatric Psychiatry*, a randomized, controlled study found that AAT is a promising option for the treatment of agitation/aggression and depression in patients with dementia. "Our results suggest that AAT may delay progression of neuropsychiatric symptoms in demented nursing home residents. Further research is needed to determine its long-term effects."

In a study performed at Mayo Clinic and published in 2015, the researchers concluded that:

- Pets enhance the quality of life of patients, especially regarding aging, cardiovascular diseases, and overall sense of wellness.

- Patients who have had a heart attack and have a companion animal, have a 5-fold increase in 1-year survival.
- Patients who are elderly and with dementia, when eating in front of a portable aquarium, have an increased lean body mass compared with patients who eat in isolation.
- The physiologic effects of petting an animal are quantifiable; they include increases in serotonin, dopamine, prolactin, and oxytocin.

> **Animal-Assisted Therapy at Mayo Clinic: The Time is Now**
>
> **Animal-Assisted Therapies and Dementia: A Systematic Mapping Review Using the Lived Environment Life Quality (LELQ) Model**

Dance Therapy

The American Dance Therapy Association states that "Dance/Movement Therapy (DMT) is the psychotherapeutic use of movement to promote emotional, social, cognitive, and physical integration of the individual, for the purpose of improving health and well-being."

> **What is Dance/Movement Therapy?**

In the journal *The Arts in Psychotherapy*, a randomized controlled trial showed promise for mitigating cognitive decline, and demonstrated how useful dance is for people who are dealing with symptoms of dementia and cognitive decline.

This recent article says, "DMT significantly improved Quality of Life, especially psychological well-being and general life in the short and long term; Social relations, Global value, and Physical health improved significantly in the short term; spirituality and general life improved in the long term as an effect of dance therapy." ("The Arts in Psychotherapy" Volume 39, Issue 4, September 2012, Pages 296-303 The efficacy of dance movement therapy group on improvement of quality of life: A randomized controlled trial, Bräuninger, I).

Light Therapy

People with Alzheimer's typically have problems with sleep, specifically sleep/wake patterns and circadian rhythms (we covered this subject under Body). We discussed how light has been used both in clinical and non-clinical settings. The summary of this research is a good read and shows that light therapy has a strong effect on various symptoms like depression and agitation, which are risk factors for Alzheimer's Disease.

> ### Light Therapy and Alzheimer's Disease and Related Dementia: Past, Present, and Future

In the May 2017 *Journal of Neurodegenerative Disease Management*, it states that "light therapy is an effective, non-pharmacological intervention in mitigating symptoms of dementia." Simple.

> ### Light, Sleep and Circadian Rhythms in Older Adults with Alzheimer's Disease and Related Dementias

Music Therapy

Music impacts portions of a person's brain, but not the areas associated with Alzheimer's disease. Music influences different senses. In this powerful video, the subject suddenly "wakes up" when he begins discussing music and its impact on him.

Man In Nursing Home Reacts To Hearing Music From His Era

Music therapy has been shown only anecdotally (largely in case studies) to be another non-pharmacological intervention that can soothe those who are agitated by the effects of Alzheimer's or dementia. Unfortunately, there is little research available and more needs to be conducted.

Music Therapy in Moderate and Severe Dementia of Alzheimer's Type: A Case-Control Study

An additional publication demonstrates the efficacy of music therapy in veterans suffering from Post-Traumatic Stress Disorder (PTSD). This paper states that "Music therapy can reduce stress, anxiety, and pain, as well as engage military members in meaningful activity as opposed to destructive thoughts or substance abuse."

Music Therapy for Post-Traumatic Stress in Adults: A Theoretical Review

Medical Cannabis

Things have certainly changed. Initially opposed to the growing and distribution of marijuana, John Boehner, former Republican Speaker of the U.S. House of Representatives, and William Weld, formerly the Republican Governor of Massachusetts, now say that "attitudes have changed."

John Boehner and Bill Weld to join

Acreage Board of Directors

Currently, cannabis is a Class 1 drug (the same as heroin). Thirty-three states (and counting) have legalized the use of medical marijuana to fight pain or treat other disease and disorders. The NIH and the National Institute on Drug Abuse still argue for more research, and we agree.

NIH Research on Marijuana and Cannabinoids

The challenges of this research are many. There are some promising breakthroughs and there is a great deal of science. Research is significant on cannabis (and CBD oil) positively influencing the negative effects of epilepsy, pain, inflammation, neuropathy, memory, anticonvulsants, and analgesics. There are over 600 abstracts of studies in the following links.

Nearly 100 Conclusions on the Health Effects of Marijuana and Cannabis-Derived Products Presented in New Report; One of the Most Comprehensive Studies of Recent Research on Health Effects of Recreational and Therapeutic Use of Cannabis and Cannabis-Derived Products

The Health Effects of Cannabis and Cannabinoids

Cannabis seems to reverse the aging processes… in the brains of mice! This is at least a start and eventually needs to be demonstrated in humans.

Cannabis Reverses Aging Processes in the Brain, Study Suggests

With Alzheimer's Disease, we see some novel therapies that may prevent the start or the progression of the disease. Cannabis is one of those therapies.

> ### Cannabis and Alzheimer's Disease: A Systematic Review of the Evidence

With Alzheimer's, the use of cannabis could also be of therapeutic value in slowing or halting certain characteristics of the disease.

> ### The Potential Therapeutic Effects of THC on Alzheimer's Disease

> ### Cannabinoids for Treatment of Alzheimer's Disease: Moving Toward the Clinic

Other articles also report and suggest that cannabis might have therapeutic potential for Alzheimer's. The use of CBD oil in combination with cannabis may be another therapy of value for the AD patient.

> ### The Therapeutic Potential of the Phytocannabinoid Cannabidiol for Alzheimer's Disease

While more research is needed, the terrible opiate epidemic may be slowed when cannabis is substituted for the opioid. Cannabis is often suggested for use in pain management.

> ### Medical Cannabis Use Is Associated With Decreased Opiate Medication Use in a Retrospective Cross-Sectional Survey of Patients With Chronic Pain

A blog from March 2017 with the headline that says, "Undeniable Evidence: Cannabis, Alzheimer's and Dementia," claims that small amounts of THC can help reduce (and in some cases even reverse) the symptoms of Alzheimer's Disease. This is a website run by medical cannabis advocates, so they may be cherry-picking the studies that they are quoting from.

Undeniable Evidence: Cannabis, Alzheimer's and Dementia

Cannabis is a controversial subject. But with the rise of dementia and increasing legalization of medical cannabis, many people will make claims about "miracles."

The best science journals and researchers know that the better studies are randomized, controlled trials, double-blind, with placebos, peer-reviewed, and published in reputable journals. Beyond that, there are longitudinal studies, i.e., studies over time. When there are similar studies, they need to be reported in the same manner. And these empirical studies should be replicable. We applaud those who are crossing boundaries to find more unique and inventive approaches to treating and responding to Alzheimer's, dementia, pain, and inflammation, and we believe more research needs to be done.

TESTS TO ASSESS AN INDIVIDUAL'S COGNITIVE DECLINE

This book is all about awareness, education, and action. The tests below do not determine whether or not you have dementia. They are free tests to help you test yourself or another person to assess cognitive decline. But they are just indicators. These tests can be helpful, and results can be useful for your doctor in interpreting results specific to your case.

Remember that the information you may derive from such tests is intended to supplement, not replace, the advice of a trained health professional. If you believe you have a health problem, it is incumbent upon you to consult a health professional. See your family physician, set up an MRI or PET Scan, along with other tests they may recommend, for a more definitive answer.

The Mini-Cog
The Montreal Cognitive Assessment (MOCA)
SAGE: A Test to Detect Signs of Alzheimer's and Dementia

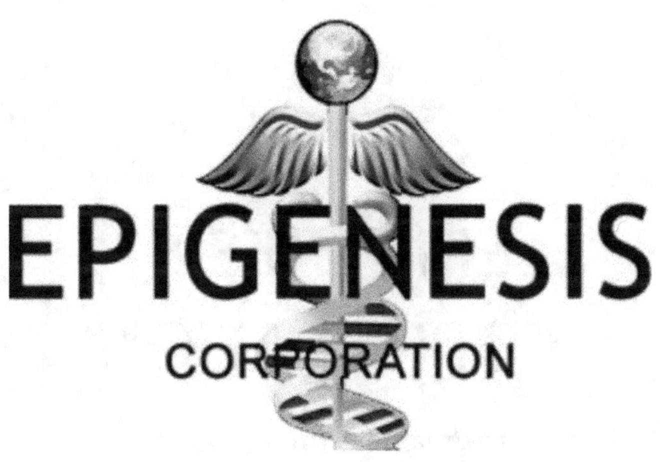
EPIGENESIS
CORPORATION

EPIGENESIS CORPORATION

Why did we build an organization to share research about how we might prevent or mitigate dementia? We wanted to summarize the best research available to take the guesswork out of what you might read on the internet. We created this via an eBook so we could continuously update the research. We then created a health and wellness coaching/consulting business and offer specific behavioral change platforms to facilitate learning and practicing lifestyle changes. Finally, we wanted to introduce you to the new science of epigenetics, for it is through behavioral coaching and epigenetics that we believe you can best create a new you!

We started with a focus on Alzheimer's Disease because it extracts a tremendous amount of money, resources, happiness, and human potential from millions of lives every day. The potential value of medical advances that delay the onset of AD could be significant.

In the "Forum for Health Economics and Policy" the authors report in a microsimulation study that from 2010 to 2050, the number of individuals ages 70+ with AD will increase 157%, from 3.6 to 9.1 million. Moreover, the annual costs associated with AD will increase from $307 billion ($181 billion formal, $126 billion informal care costs) to $1.5 trillion. The authors take data samples from the Health and Retirement Study (1998-2008) and the Aging Demographics and Memory Study. The authors state that if we could delay the onset of AD by five years, it would result in 41% lower prevalence and 40% lower cost, 2.7 additional life years (about 5 AD-free), and a cost savings of $511,208 per person.

The Value of Delaying Alzheimer's Disease Onset

The question to be addressed by Epigenesis Corporation is this: Can an evidence-based, non-invasive, non-pharmacological protocol encompassing body, environment, emotion, mindfulness, and spirituality delay the onset of Alzheimer's disease or other forms of dementia? We believe it can make a difference. To that end, we have created Epigenesis IP, LLC; Epigenesiscorp.com where you can purchase additional copies of this book, access our caregiver's forum, and stay up to date on all the latest research about dementia and cognitive decline.

Epigenesiscorp.com

Confronting Alzheimer's

Implications are that delaying the onset of AD would reduce economic impact, increase longevity, and mitigate the deleterious effects on those suffering from AD, their families, caregivers, and organizations.

BEEMS

BEEMS is Epigenesis Corporation's new health and wellness approach that invokes aspects of body, emotion, environment, mindfulness, and spirituality in order to alter this debilitating, costly, and progressive disease. As previously stated in this eBook, **B** represents the <u>Body</u>, including exercise, sleep, lifelong learning, and nutrition; **E** represents <u>Emotion</u>, such as anger and depression, and modeling "grace under pressure." **E** also represents the <u>Environment</u>, including the air we breathe, friends in our world, and the place where we live; **M** represents <u>Mindfulness,</u> including being present, mindful, and meditative; and **S** represents our <u>Spirituality</u>, that is, a belief in a higher power, God perhaps, or the best and highest good of mankind.

In this eBook, we examine the evidenced-based research for dementia with a special emphasis on epigenetics, a new science that allows us to "switch on and switch off" genetic markers that may represent, enable, and disable the onset of this terrible disease.

Here are a few summary ideas from the **BEEMS** protocol you may want to try:

- Get up and move 20 minutes every day;
- Take supplements that complement, such as gingko Biloba, turmeric/curcumin, and fish oil (DHA);
- Pay attention to what you use for cooking your foods (avoid aluminum);
- Pay attention to what you store your food in (glass is best);

- Try to get 7-8 hours of sleep every night;
- Avoid processed foods and especially sugar;
- Meditate, breathe deeply, and cleanse;
- Think and keep an active mind; and
- Eat well and love your neighbors and your friends!

All of these actions can activate your BDNF (Brain-Derived Neurotrophic Factor). This influences DNA and catalyzes DNA to produce more BDNF, which protects brain neurons. This can mitigate susceptibility to and the rapid onset of AD.

We said earlier that several studies, e.g., the Nun Study, the FINGER Study, and the China Study, inform us about how and what to use as interventions for mitigating cognitive decline and for helping change behavior. Here we offer even more evidence to demonstrate that we are in alignment with some of the best research available to the public.

The *Journal of Alzheimer's and Dementia* published a summary of the evidence on modifiable risk factors for cognitive decline and dementia in June of 2015. The results underscore the relevance of the BEEMS protocol. In this article, conclusions summarize the strength of evidence concerning risk factors for cognitive decline. Also shown is the strength of evidence concerning risk factors for dementia.

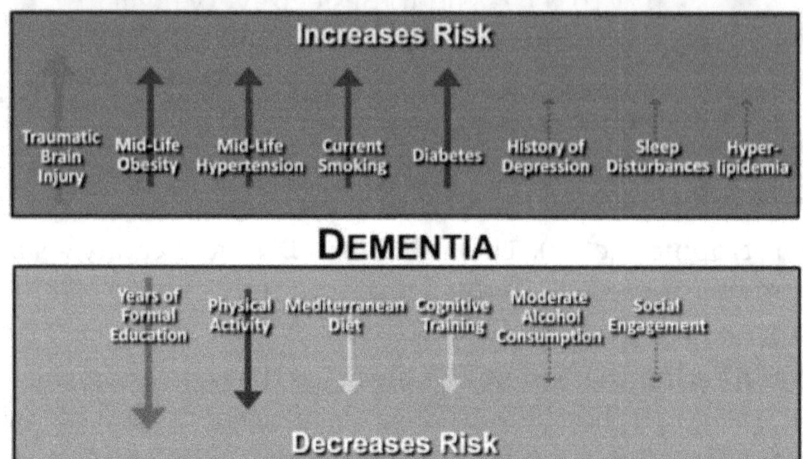

> ## Summary of the Evidence on Modifiable Risk Factors for Cognitive Decline and Dementia: A Population-based Perspective

The results of the FINGER study reinforce those from the summary in the *Journal of Alzheimer's and Dementia*. This consistency in results suggests that there are a multivariate set of approaches to reducing one's risk for getting some form of dementia.

> ## A 2 Year Multidomain Intervention of Diet, Exercise, Cognitive Training, and Vascular Risk Monitoring versus Control to Prevent Cognitive Decline in At-Risk Elderly People (FINGER): a Randomised Controlled Trial

> ## Inside the FINGER Study: Hard Evidence Shows How Diet, Exercise and Mind Games Might Make or Break a Dementia Diagnosis

In the FINGER Study, much like the upcoming POINTER Study, the investigators recognized that a systems and holistic approach that leverages lifestyle and non-invasive factors, versus a vaccine or tablet/pill approach, is likely to give us a way to lessen cognitive decline and reduce our chances of becoming demented. Not surprisingly, this approach also has positive outcomes for diabetes, cardiovascular disease, and cancer.

U.S. Study to Protect Brain Health Through Lifestyle Intervention to Reduce Risk (POINTER)

The U.S. Alzheimer's Association is launching a new brain health education program called "Healthy Habits for a Healthier You," with a goal similar to what we have suggested in this eBook to help you take better care of your bodies and brains. We believe that with this information, not only can you become better informed, but you also can have a more useful and open dialogue with your primary care physician.

Additionally, we are calling for a Framingham-type study for dementia. Developing a longitudinal, epidemiological set of data that can be examined and used by multiple researchers is a part of the "gold standard" for any evidence-based study.

Framingham Heart Study (FHS)

The Institute of Medicine and the National Academies of Sciences, Engineering and Medicine reinforced what the U.S. Alzheimer's Association has advocated with the Institute of Medicine's book, *Cognitive Aging: Progress in Understanding and Opportunities for Action*. Exercise, not smoking, weight control, social activity, and lifelong learning are all things that can reduce the risk of cognitive decline and perhaps the risk of dementia.

However, more research and resources are needed—especially

more longitudinal, multi-factor, population-based, and randomized controlled trials – to determine the specific set of interventions that will make us a healthier nation. This is a public health policy issue and represents a campaign for our future.

For nearly 20 years, Dr. Barry Spiker has studied the value of the mature worker and the contribution the mature worker has in the organization. Losing older workers' wisdom, presence, productivity, and contributions is a loss to organizations, society, and the workers' personal growth. Overall it is a terrible loss of human capital! Epigenesis Corporation has established a management consulting practice to address these issues.

Establishing the Positive Contributory Value of Older Workers: A Positive Psychology Perspective

The possible impact of new evidence-based protocol could have a far-reaching and demonstrable impact on Alzheimer's prevention and treatment, as well as economic savings and cost avoidance for individuals, organizations, society, and healthcare at large. The impact of dementia on organizations is discussed in the next section. We also discuss a relatively new concept, "The Caring Company."

HEALTH AND WELLNESS COACHING

There is an emerging consensus as to what is referred to as health and wellness coaching—namely, it is a patient-centered process that is based upon behavior change theory and delivered by health professionals. Our approach is not much different from this definition, and there is so much more we can add by focusing on Body, Emotion, Environment, Mindfulness, and Spirituality (BEEMS).

Change is hard. In Dr. Dale Bredesen's book, *The End of Alzheimer's: The First Program to Prevent and Reverse Cognitive Decline*, 2017, he acknowledges this when quoting Machiavelli:

> It must be remembered that there is nothing more difficult to plan, more doubtful of success, nor more dangerous to manage than a new system. For the initiator has the enmity of all who would profit by the preservation of the old institution and merely lukewarm defenders in those who gain by the new one.

CHAPTER 12 OF DR. BREDESEN'S BOOK BEGINS WITH THE ABOVE QUOTE BUT SAYS VERY LITTLE ABOUT HOW TO ACHIEVE POSITIVE BEHAVIORAL CHANGE. WE OFFER A UNIQUE PROGRAM (BEEMS) WITH PH.D.S IN BEHAVIORAL CHANGE THAT IS RELATIVELY

COST-EFFECTIVE AND IS RELATIVELY EASY FOR AN INDIVIDUAL TO IMPLEMENT. WE OFFER MANY INSIGHTS ON HOW TO CHANGE BEHAVIOR, REINFORCED WITH COACHING FROM EXPERTS IN BEHAVIORAL CHANGE, PRIMARILY PH.D.S.

There are many kinds of dementia. Our focus is on the behaviors that might lead to dementia, and specifically those behaviors that could be moderated, mitigated, or stopped completely. Dementia is not a "one-size fits all" type of problem. Again we want to emphasize that if you are experiencing symptoms that make you think you may be on a path toward dementia, speak with your family medical doctor.

THE PLATFORMS OF BEHAVIORAL CHANGE

Here we want to provide you more information on what we mean by coaching for behavioral change. First, what do we mean by health and wellness coaching?

Health coaches help you target behavioral changes and set goals for your specific health-related outcomes. They help with education, motivation, self-awareness, and identifying specific tasks or skills linked to outcomes that are measurable and determinative. Health coaches are there to support and guide you towards healthier outcomes. They help you find your internal strengths and link those with external resources to create sustainable change. It is a systemic process!

Here is a summary review of health coaching and a review of the scientific literature which offers some operational definitions of what health and wellness coaching is about. The coaching business is currently inconsistent and is calling out for standardization. Its most important feature, however, is that it is a personalized approach. One size will not fit all, and so we come to the coaching experience with a methodology that strongly supports a personalized experience.

Health Coaching: Another Component of Personalized Medicine for Patients with Chronic Obstructive Pulmonary Disease

A Systematic Review of the Literature on

Health and Wellness Coaching: Defining a Key Behavioral Intervention in Healthcare

---

Alcoholics Anonymous and Smoker's Nicotine Anonymous

The two most public and personal behavioral change programs center on alcohol and smoking. Moreover, they are "complementary behaviors," and while smoking cessation and drinking behaviors are not the focus of this eBook, both are implicated in dementia and in lifestyle/behavioral coaching. AA says its success rate ranged in the upward 30th percentile for smoking cessation in the years between 1965 and 2010. The rates for alcohol abstinence are all over the place, from 5% to 75%. In addressing both behaviors, counseling or coaching and support groups are used. Our dementia prevention protocol adopts some of the same principals as are prevalent in AA and smoking cessation programs.

Smoking and Drinking as Complementary Behaviors
Alcohol Alert: Alcohol and Tobacco
What Defines Success in Alcoholics Anonymous?
Quitting Smoking Among Adults --- United States, 2001--2010

Brief Therapy

Brief therapy is just as it sounds—brief, i.e., generally ten sessions or as many as 20. It is designed to help people manage a specific problem or make a single desired change. It is focused on the present – the here and now. Typically, it is about solving a current problem, and most therapists take a cognitive-behavioral (CBT) approach to helping the client solve their specific problem.

Solution-Focused Brief Therapy

Cognitive-Behavioral Therapy

In Cognitive-Behavioral Therapy (CBT), the focus is on solving problems, goal setting, and achievement of a goal. The therapist/coach helps the client focus on beliefs, assumptions, and behaviors that they want to change. The client is challenged to make healthier choices and free themselves from negative emotional states and patterns of unhelpful behavior based on faulty thinking, thus enabling them to make healthier choices.

Cognitive-Behavioral Therapies: Achievements and Challenges

Dialectical Behavior Therapy

Initially developed in the late 1980s by Dr. Marsha Linnehan to treat borderline personality disorder, Dialectical Behavior Therapy (DBT) extends upon CBT and emphasizes the psychosocial aspects of treatment. It focuses on the intensity of emotions driving the feelings, attitudes, and beliefs of an individual. For borderlines, emotions are very strong and are often black and white, suggesting that clients may not be equipped with the skills necessary to deal with surges of emotion. For these individuals, a therapist and often a team of therapists attempt to inculcate new skills around four things:

1. Mindfulness
2. Interpersonal Effectiveness
3. Distress Tolerance

4. Emotional Regulation

"Radical acceptance" is a pretty strong expression, yes? This idea can help you tolerate distress. Marsha Linnehan (1993a) coined the term and suggests that this is the first step toward changing your life. It starts with a change in attitude, acknowledging your present situation without being critical of yourself, and accepting the situation in the here and now without blaming yourself or others. Simply accept *what is* and plan to move forward. Focus your attention on what you can do right now.

Dialectical Behavior Therapy is, as Dr. Linnehan has said, building who you are for "a life worth living."

An Overview of Dialectical Behavior Therapy

Neuro-Linguistic Programming

Neuro-Linquistic Programming (NLP) is often called "the language of the mind," with a goal of building alignment between the unconscious and conscious parts of your mind. It can be referred to as learning to "walk the talk." Watch this brief video and examine the content.

So, What Is NLP?

Results on the effectiveness of NLP are mixed, but for some people it is an easy way to change thought patterns or behaviors.

What Is NLP and What Is It Used for?

Psych-K

Dr. Bruce Lipton and Rob Williams are experts both in epigenetics and in changing one's belief system that culminates in changing behavior. We offer this information to familiarize you with one very successful approach that is easily implemented. Rob Williams shares how he leads people to behavioral change in this YouTube video.

Rob Williams The Psychology of Change Bruce Lipton

Psych-K is based upon applied kinesiology (muscle testing) and is practiced by many clinicians and individuals. It is easy to learn and can help you change your behavior.

Question: What is PSYCH-K?

DEMENTIA'S IMPACT ON ORGANIZATIONS

In the Wisconsin Department of Health Services's article, "The Impact of Caregivers in the Workplace," we read:

Employees with caregiving responsibilities are faced with competing obligations and increased stress. A study by the Metlife Mature Market Institute estimated the cost to U.S. companies in lost productivity, absenteeism, disengagement, turnover, and increased healthcare costs for fulltime employed caregivers is as much as $34 billion a year. That equates to $2,110 for every fulltime employee who cares for an adult.

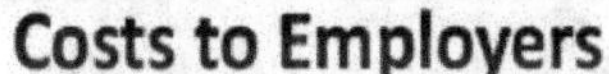

Costs to Employers

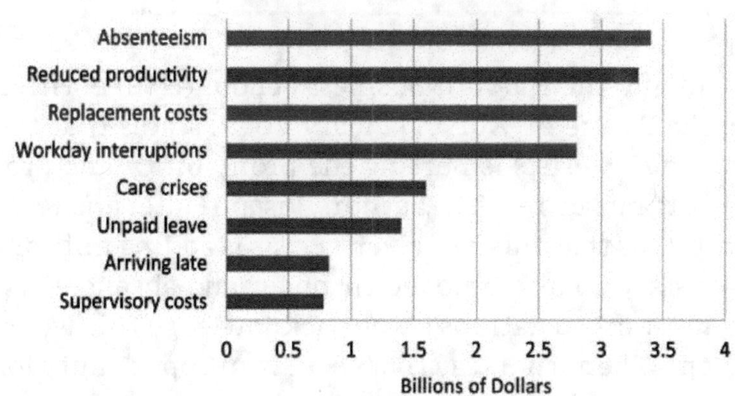

And further, the article states that:

Potential benefits of becoming a dementia-friendly employer and being a solutions provider include:

- Attracting and retaining the best workers;
- Preserving the historical knowledge and experience of seasoned employees by keeping them in the workplace;
- Reducing the costs of recruiting, hiring, and training new employees;
- Reducing health insurance costs;
- Experiencing less absenteeism and fewer disruptions in work schedules;
- Improving productivity, morale, and engagement;
- Enhancing positive image and reputation in the community;
- Remaining competitive;
- Having fewer accidents related to employee stress;
- Simplifying the ability to locate and find resources.

The Impact of Caregivers in the Workplace

A recent study by the Harvard Business School (HBS) entitled "Managing the Future of Work," January 2019, states that the growing caregiving crisis is hurting the profitability and productivity of organizations. The authors, Joseph Fuller and Manjari Raman, tell us that this caregivers' crisis is adding millions in hidden costs such as employee turnover and absenteeism. Worse yet, most organizations do not acknowledge this workplace problem. The authors say that there is an opportunity for organizations to implement a "care strategy" to better support their employees. We could not agree more.

The Caring Company

When a spouse or parent begins to show the symptoms of dementia, be it Alzheimer's, Parkinson's, or some other form of cognitive disorder, organizations do not necessarily respond in a caring fashion, nor do they allow for their employees to better manage their time and resources to provide caregiving *and* take care of themselves. A legitimate question for any organization is reflected in the article, "Employee Eldercare Responsibilities: Should Organizations Care?" The HBS study asks the following: 1) Are there enough employees with eldercare concerns to warrant organizational intervention? 2) What types of eldercare arrangements are typical, and how satisfactory are these arrangements? 3) How do eldercare responsibilities affect caregivers as they assume the role of an organizational employee?

**Employee Eldercare Responsibilities:
Should Organizations Care?**

Specifically, how are eldercare responsibilities related to caregivers' job attitudes and job behaviors such as absenteeism and intent to quit?

Finally, do employees, both those who have eldercare responsibilities and those who do not have current eldercare concerns, support organizationally-sponsored eldercare benefits? We know that often the best employees can quit and find work elsewhere, and turnover largely impacts women's participation in the workforce. Thus, critical knowledge often leaves the organization, especially in organizations where no knowledge capture methodology is in place. An organization often suffers because of retention issues, and can suffer because of reputational issues that can emerge if an organization comes to be known as one that does not care about its employees.

One of the authors of this eBook had an accident and sought assistance or accommodation from their organization. However, as this occurred in a "work at will" state, the organization was limited in terms of what it could do. The organization could not give time off to the employee to partake in therapy unless that employee took a pay cut. Moreover, a pay cut was not feasible because of the out-of-pocket costs associated with additional care.

The employee was fearful of taking a leave of absence, because, again, being in an "at-will" state, the employee thought they then would become a "target" for future dismissal. Disability was not an answer either for the very same reason. Our colleague was eventually let go in a small layoff, ironically after the company's Human Resources head had received letters from health care professionals indicating a need for time off for the employee. It could be said that this organization did not have a caring culture, and everyone lost with this move: the company, the customers, and the employee.

The authors at Harvard suggest that organizations become *Caring Companies* and find ways to help their employees when tragedy strikes at home. There are a host of ways an organization can address the "care crisis" and reap the benefits.

First, in order to retain talent, organizations can help facilitate those employees who are caregivers. Often the best employees are the ones who can and will leave if the organization does not support them. Talent retention has organization-wide benefits, e.g., knowledge retention, mentoring younger and less experienced employees, as well as all other advantages related to what has been called Knowledge Management.

Knowledge Management (KM) is a way to share information collected across the organization. It helps an organization make better decisions, inculcates a culture of organizational learning, enables collaboration and cooperation, increases productivity, enables reuse of existing skills, and positions the organization to be better able to compete and benchmark with other employers in their particular business sector. This is not just another business benefit, but should be seen through a lens of improving an organization's top line *and* bottom line.

Second, organizations can demonstrate a commitment to a culture of caring. This is a way of engendering employee engagement and employee loyalty. An employee who is engaged believes they are valued and will always find innovative ways to solve problems and be a part of the decision-making process. A loyal employee is the first line of defense and is the best free marketing any organization can enjoy. The loyal employee goes above and beyond and is forever passionate about what they do. There is simply no good way to monetize those behaviors—you recognize it when it happens. Some other benefits of being a culture of caring are enhanced decision-making, greater creativity, and more innovation.

Finally, organizations can measure employees' attitudes toward the corporate/organizational culture. As is so often the case, what gets measured gets done, and what gets done gets rewarded. This applies to employees, the organization, and all outside stakeholders.

CAREGIVING AND CAREGIVERS

Part of the impetus for the eBook and this section of the eBook came from a relationship we have been fortunate to have had over the years with a mentor and friend named Jerre. His mother died from AD, and his father died of a heart attack while trying to care for her. We honor him and his family for supporting healing at all ages, and for helping to find a cure for Alzheimer's Disease.

Much has been written and studied on caregiving and its effects, e.g., financial, psychological, emotional, physical, and societal. Caring for those who are suffering from some form of dementia impacts caregivers, patients, families, and society.

Juggling Life, Work, and Caregiving

Healthcare systems are overwhelmed with the sheer numbers of patients, lack of adequate facilities, lack of availability of caregivers, shortages in healthcare providers, and increasing costs.

In June 2011, MetLife published a study of caregiving costs to working caregivers, and it is compelling. Here is a summary of their key findings:

- The percentage of adult children providing personal care and/or financial assistance to a parent has more than tripled over the past 15 years. Currently, a quarter of adult children, mainly Baby Boomers, provide these types of care to a parent.

- The total estimated aggregate lost wages, pensions, and Social Security benefits of these caregivers of parents is nearly $3 trillion.
- For women, the total individual amount of lost wages due to leaving the labor force early because of caregiving responsibilities equals $142,693. The estimated impact of caregiving on lost Social Security benefits is $131,351.
- A very conservative estimated impact on pensions is approximately $50,000. Thus, in total, the cost impact of caregiving on the individual female caregiver in terms of lost wages, pensions, and Social Security benefits equals $324,044.
- For men, the total individual amount of lost wages due to leaving the labor force early because of caregiving responsibilities equals $89,107. The estimated impact of caregiving on lost Social Security benefits is $144,609.
- Adding in a conservative estimate of the impact on pensions at $50,000, the total impact equals $283,716 for men and $303,880 for the average (male or female) caregiver 50+ who cares for a parent.
- Working and non-working adult children are almost equally as likely to provide care to parents in need.
- Overall, caregiving sons and daughters provide comparable care in many respects, but daughters are more likely to provide basic care, and sons are more likely to provide financial assistance.
- Adult children 50+ who work and provide care to a parent are more likely to have fair or poor health than those who do not provide care to their parents.

Assessing the long-term financial impact of caregiving for aging parents on the caregivers, especially those who must curtail their working careers to do so, is especially significant because it can jeopardize their future financial secur-

ity.
("The MetLife Study of Caregiving Costs to Working Caregivers: Double Jeopardy for Baby Boomers Caring for Their Parents," June 2011)

> ## The MetLife Study of Caregiving Costs to Working Caregivers

There is also evidence that caregivers experience considerable health issues, such as depression and anxiety, because of their focus on caring for others. In 2002, Stanford University studied the effects on family caregivers for dementia. Stunningly, they found that 40% of caregivers died from stress-related disorders before the person they were caring for had died.

> ## Stanford Study Focuses on Effects of Family Caregiving for Patients with Alzheimer's Disease and Dementia

This study, published in the *Journal of Gerontological Social Work,* addresses the issue of who cares for the caregiver.

> ## Who Cares for Caregivers? Evidence-based Approaches to Family Support

The following article from *Time Magazine* amplifies even more significant problems with the costs of caregiving and studies the few states that are trying to prepare for this demographical doom.

> ## A Growing American Crisis: Who Will Care for the Baby Boomers?

The need for flexibility in the workplace and policies that benefit working caregivers is likely to increase in importance as more working caregivers approach their retirement while still caring for an aging parent. We cover this issue in greater detail in the section on Dementia's Impact on Organizations.

Caregiving Resources

There are many caregiver resources available on the Internet. We will not attempt to aggregate and curate everything, but rather will offer some of the best material we found. Recommendations from the Alzheimer's Foundation of America is a good start.

- **Educate yourself about the disease.** A variety of valuable information concerning Alzheimer's disease and related illnesses can be found on our website under support groups, educational workshops, and utilizing community resources and professionals. These sources will also increase your knowledge of the disease and what to expect.
- **Build your skills.** Key skills for any care partner include communication, understanding safety considerations, understanding behaviors, and managing activities of daily living.
- **Develop empathy.** It is important to gain an understanding of what it is like to be a person living with dementia, experiencing this loss, while recognizing your losses. Manage your expectations of your loved one and remain patient with the disease.
- **Avoid caregiver burnout.** Make time for yourself! Seek support (and there are many community support groups), eat well, get sleep, exercise, and focus on you!
- **Support is critical.** Seek support from family, friends, and medical and mental health professionals. They can assist you when things get tough.
- **Stay active & engaged.** Be mindful of what brings your loved one pleasure so they may maintain an active and meaningful life, whether this is through exercise, entertainment, music, or the arts.
- **Advocate.** Be involved in your loved one's medical care. Know who the care team members are, ask questions, ex-

press concerns, and discuss treatment options.

- **Be prepared.** Take care of financial, legal, and long-term care planning issues. Try to involve your loved one in decision-making if they are still capable and consider their wishes related to future care and end of life issues.
- **Do not forget to connect.** Kindness, humor, and creativity are essential parts of caregiving. Hugs, gentle touch, and compassion will help your loved one feel connected and loved.
- **Stay positive.** Focus on the capabilities and strengths that remain with your loved one and enjoy your relationship while you are still together. (https://alzfdn.org/caregiving-resources/)

Alzheimer's Foundation of America

The National Council on Aging started in 1950 and is a leading voice and advocate for older Americans. Many resources are free and easily available to the caregiver.

National Council on Aging

We also like the National Alliance for Caregiving and the Caregiver Action Network.

Caregiving Organization
Caregiver Action Network

The National Family Caregiver's Association is another resource that advocates for the nearly "50 million Americans who care for the chronically ill, aged or disabled loved one."

National Family Caregivers Association (NFCA)

In the following report, the AARP (always a good resource) discusses what the caregiver industry outlook currently is and will be in the very near future. You can download this free report. It will give you a sense of just how large and growing the caregiver business is.

Finally, but certainly not exhaustive, is information from the American Society on Aging. The society lists on their website 25 organizations that take care of caregivers.

Caregiving Innovation Frontiers

25 Organizations that Take Care of Caregivers

After one of our colleagues had a major heart attack, they sat down and did a thorough examination and inventory of their life. They shed weight, moved to the country, filed for a divorce, grew their own organic food, entertained friends and family, meditated, walked 3 miles every day, and got right with spirit. Seven years later, they are still enjoying what was believed to be a health breakthrough. That is our hope for you.

Reading this eBook and examining all the links to other sources is a start to taking responsibility for your own health. You are embracing possibilities for healing yourself. This is not the beginning of the end, but the end of the beginning.

LIFE IS FRAGILE AND SHORT

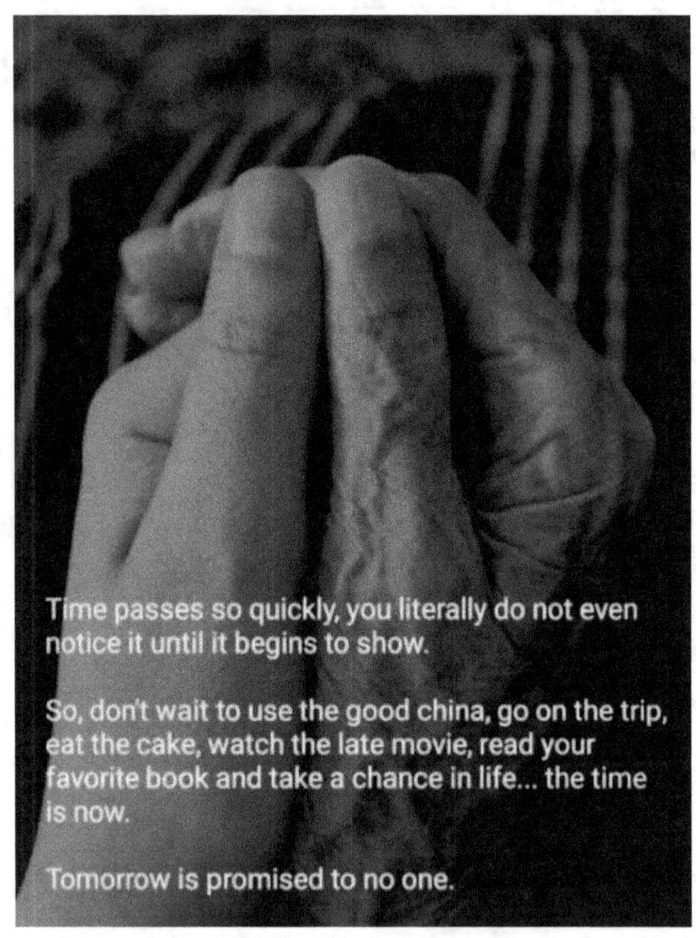

AUTHORS

BARRY K. SPIKER, PH.D.

The lead author, Barry K. Spiker, Ph.D., has published eight books, five book chapters, and several refereed articles. He has been a keynote presenter at major conferences and participated as an invited panelist at several more conferences focused on aging.

As a dissertation mentor, Barry has directed the doctoral dissertations of nearly 100 students and published over 100 academic and trade publications. Most recently, he has conducted research in aging, and has spent the last decade examining nearly all the published evidence on dementia and epigenetics. Barry is the Founder of Epigenesis IP, LLC, a benefit and conscious organization focused on coaching and supporting individuals who have concerns over becoming demented.

As a senior executive, change agent, and entrepreneur, Barry has been acknowledged internationally for his groundbreaking efforts in driving the behavioral and cultural change that builds organizational and personal effectiveness, increased revenue growth, cost savings and customer satisfaction.

As a researcher/writer, award-winning platform speaker, and facilitator, Barry is considered an expert in strategy, the value of the mature worker, human capital management, sustainability, executive development, large-scale post-merger integration, and corporate consulting. His experience spans start-ups, government, higher education, NGOs, mature companies, mergers/acquisitions, and business turnarounds. His personal center of influence consists of a network of accomplished leaders and innovators across diverse corporate and public sector cultures. His 40+ year career reflects success in the corporate world, academia, and entrepreneurship, including several years as an executive with a prestigious strategy firm and two Big Four firms.

You may contact Barry at https://www.epigenesiscorp.com or call/text at 480-721-7308.

ELIOT JEKOWSKY, PH.D., MD, MBA

Eliot has more than 30 years of experience in healthcare, as a provider and as a medical director for a large health insurance company. He studied protein synthesis in prokaryotes at M.I.T. leading to a Ph.D. in biochemistry, followed by a postdoctoral fellowship in clinical chemistry at New England Deaconess Hospital in Boston, MA. He was the Assistant Director of Clinical Chemistry at Massachusetts General Hospital in Boston, MA, for two years before pursuing more clinically-related interests by enrolling in the University of Miami Ph.D. to M.D. program, where he obtained an M.D. degree in two years. This was followed by an internship and residency in primary care internal medicine at Cambridge Hospital, an affiliate of the Harvard Medical School. After completing his residency and becoming board certified in internal medicine, he began practicing emergency medicine, eventually obtaining board certification in that specialty as well. He worked full time as a staff ED physician and held an Associate Director position.

Dr. Jekowsky enrolled in an executive M.B.A. program while continuing to practice, receiving an M.B.A. in High Technology from Northeastern University. This led to an opportunity to join a health insurance company in Rhode Island as a physician reviewer, and then to a position as a medical director at an insurer in Massachusetts. He recently retired from the position of Medical Director for Medical Policy and Medicare Advantage. As a result of his training and experience, Dr. Jekowsky has a broad view of the clinical needs for medical testing and treatments, the science behind the tests and procedures in genomic medicine, and knowledge of the business processes required for successfully bringing products to market.

COLLEEN HUNSAKER, D.O.

Colleen holds degrees in Physics & Biology with honors from the University of Pittsburgh. Following Medical School in West Virginia and additional postgraduate training in California, she served as a Naval Medical Officer and worked in the challenging field of Emergency Medicine for nearly twenty years. Upon leaving the Navy as a Lieutenant Commander, she continued in this field, working in inner-city Los Angeles for many years as an attending staff physician and also as an Assistant Director. She later worked as an ER physician in Hawaii for six years. She became a Board-Certified Fellow in Emergency Medicine in 1991 and holds certification in Diving and Hyperbaric Medicine as well.

As her interest in administration and health law started to grow, she chaired the Committee on Emergency Medical Services for LA County and was the delegate to the California Medical Association, where issues included funding for the treatment of indigent patients, disaster preparedness, specialty coverage in trauma centers, and issues related to COBRA and EMTALA.

During her extensive career as an emergency medicine physician she saw and studied the devastating effects of aging, many caused by lack of self-care, lack of preventive medical care or no medical care at all, or a lack of knowledge about the aging process and the incredible advances that have been made in this field. She then entered into the extensive field of anti-aging medicine and integrative medicine, utilizing the best of conventional medicine combined with natural alternatives and multiple spiritual modalities that have a very strong influence on health and well-being. She is also a Diplomate of the American Board of Anti-Aging and Regenerative Medicine.

Currently, Dr. Hunsaker is a principal investigator in an ongoing clinical trial related to the immune response. She is an avid equestrian fan and former competitive rider. She has one son, Todd, who, after completing his post-baccalaureate studies in Neuroscience with honors, then completed a Fulbright scholarship, studying Neuroimaging in Germany. He is currently working at Stanford in Neuroscience.

ACKNOWLEDGMENTS

My father loved to garden, as do I. He taught me about composting, readying the soil, choosing the seed, nurturing the plants as they grew. Our bodies are like a garden, and we must nourish ourselves in similar ways by feeding and fueling, creating a healthy environment early to grow in, and taking care of pests or invaders when we first are exposed to outside forces in the environment.

Life is a lot like gardening and living a full life is a lot like farming. And where would we be in this world without the farmer -- for farmers are the caretakers of the earth and are the metaphor for our caregivers. To that end we want to acknowledge and honor the importance of caretakers and caregivers of those who are suffering with dementia. The world needs people who will help us all thrive, and this begins with a commitment from each human being to do what it takes to effectively nurture themselves and then, one another.

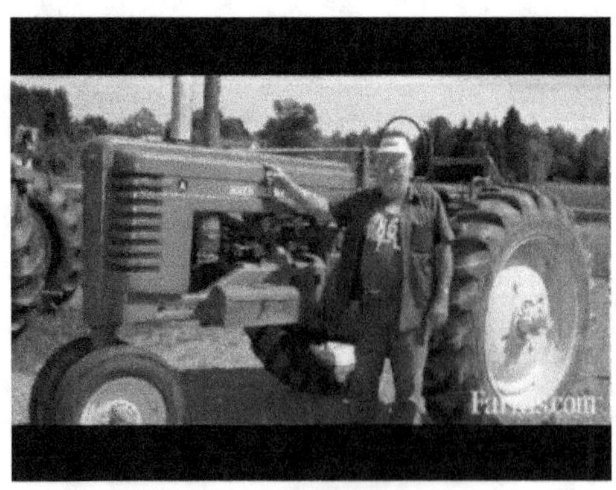

As many of us age and our health declines, we become increasingly dependent on others to help us. Whether family or friends or paid caregivers, that is a tough job; some say it is the world's toughest job. Some are paid, but most caregivers are not. As a society we have a duty, a responsibility to care for our aging population.

As the numbers of the aging increase, many in ill health and suffering from cognitive decline, it should be a wakeup call to all policymakers and leaders that this is the time to come together and focus on solutions. How will we assist those who have little money and maybe few loved ones to care for them as they get older? What if we suddenly find we have no caretakers, no caregivers, and no one is left with us to face the pain, sadness, and uncertainty of what futures we have left? How can we do that to ourselves, our neighbors, our communities?

We cannot fathom that possibility. And so we need to look at the potential options and solutions that are out there. Fortunately for this eBook project, we have had the incredible talents, passions, energy, and intellects of so many people who contributed by sharing a part of themselves.

First, Dr. Paul Coleman, whose passion for Alzheimer's research got Barry interested in dementia seven years ago, and who has done research over nearly 70 years that is truly groundbreaking and pathfinding. Paul should be considered the "grandfather" of Alzheimer's research. He is already transitioning Dr. Diego Mastroeni, a colleague at ASU Biodesign Institute, to move forward, along with others in his research lab as they work to develop a blood test to determine very early if an individual has dementia.

Dianne Price, a friend and the former head of communications at ASU Biodesign, and who made sure Paul and Diego's research gets out there (along with that of 150 other incredible faculty and researchers) and is distributed to the public. Then there is Dr. Sheri Crain, who reminded me to re-read Dr. Bruce Lipton's book, "The Biology of Belief," back nearly 10 years ago, and inspired the beginnings of Epigenesis; and Mead Rose, who died in my arms as our webmaster seven years ago and has never left my heart. Mead also introduced us to Michelle Pate, another healer, coach, and intellect who has been through it all.

There is Carla Carter, long-time friend and colleague who is a quality guru and process management czar and a dear friend of nearly 40 years yet still invites me out to lunch and dinner; Drs. Larry and Verna Wangler, who read and reviewed several original copies of the book, making excellent suggestions for the everyday reader, and always found time for us while going through family health challenges themselves.

Ramona Melvin, an alternative healer from North Carolina, who introduced me to Mead (and her former husband, Russell Wright, who believed curation was king and saw that embedded links would provide access to original sources).

And there are my co-authors, especially Dr. Colleen Hunsaker (and her son Todd), whose concern and careful observations about my health encouraged me to seek several diagnostics after suffering a fall and what eventually was diagnosed as a traumatic brain injury – she is an indispensable colleague and our 1st Chief Medical Officer, Board Certified in Integrative Medicine, Emergency Medicine and a Diplomate in Aging. There is Dr. Eliot Jekowsky, one of the smartest individuals I have ever met, always with a kind word, always gathering newly published material to make us more current and approachable for our readers, and who wrestled all my notes into something intelligible about the "Body."

Dr. John Wyrick, who introduced me to Eliot (EJ) and brings spirit and light to all that we do; and cherished friend, Laura Brown, who co-authored with me and introduced me to Dr. John; the Brain Alliance folks in Arizona and in every state; the Area Agencies on Aging (the front lines and all the state-run Advisory Councils on Aging; and the Osher Learning Institutes, honoring all life-long learning and the building of cognitive reserve); the U.S. and World Alzheimer's Associations; and the U.S. and World Dementia organizations and the World Health Organization.

Linda Levitt, who facilitated the latest meaning-making of this eBook and gave of herself with no expectation of remuneration, but because she was seeking a nobler purpose, worked her tail off and kicked my rear-end to get this eBook done; and fine artist Mary Linda Mills of Durango, a very special lady, who painted the cover from the heart and all of the inside covers from the elucidation of her spirit and the bright, colorful and meaningful elements that she sees and envisions; and then there are all the folks who met in Sedona nearly four years ago to help plan this business, who gave of themselves, financially and spiritually (26 people); and that just scratches the surface.

The folks in Sedona came together for 2+ days in January 2016, laughed, talked, played music, shared stories of how they met Barry, broke bread, slept by Oak Creek, and yet stayed on point, giving us a roadmap for where we should go and how best to get there.

It was four years ago; today it seems like an eternity ago, but it also has streamed by so quickly. We shall never forget Joan Rall, "retired" from being a Partner at Ernst and Young, who traveled from her homes in New York and Massachusetts, served admirably as one of our first Board Members, helped us with our spreadsheets and what kinds of investments we would need.

Mike Harrison, dear friend and also legal savant, business advisor, coach, consultant, friend, and truly a remarkable human being who plays a mean banjo and guitar; and Dennis Egan, another individual who believed in what we were doing, friend of nearly 50 years and legal barrister who always knew exactly and precisely what the right words should be, and who is the former captain of my debate team back in Marquette, Michigan; also from Northern Michigan University is Patrick Theut (soon to be a Ph.D.) and his partner, Dr. Roxanna Transit, who drafted our first Private Placement Memorandum.

Benjamin Spiker, who introduced us to the concept of financial gerontology while an executive at Merrill-Lynch, who now is entrepreneur and owner of the Investment Management Group (Shore to Summit), and who brought his colleague, Christopher Jensen, another attorney in Baltimore (and we could not have enough individuals like CJ who introduced us to the VC world).

Michelle Muller (aka, the *Hempress*), dear friend and colleague, mother of 4 amazing young adults, who launched her own business in CBD oil and uncovered cannabinoid research that was originally unknown to us, and who is currently helping people who are already afflicted with this horrific disease.

Then there are the rest of our medical docs: Dr. Steve Cruikshank, North Carolina, OBGYN then Board Certified in Oncology and Integrative Medicine; Dr. Don Miller, Prescott, AZ, first an orthopedic doc (and team doc to many professional sports teams) and an early student of CTE and TBI, now an attorney working with vets to help them get what they need after their service; and Dr. David Sellen, Los Angeles, CA, who died while waiting for a lung transplant, but did yeoman's work in implementing an epigenetic intervention to keep his med students in their 4th year of medical school while he did his 3rd doctorate with Barry – may God bless him as he will be sorely missed.

Dr. Hollie Koppel, another doctoral student, who uncovered the leadership secrets from superstar leaders who used an epigenetic platform; Ken Whiting, always the altruist and always the first to grab a check; Ted Coonfield, former Board Member, personal and professional advisor, amazing chef, close friend of over 40 years and straight talker...nothing could be better; Glenn Graham, another former Board Member, soft-spoken, intellectual, Harley owner and gun enthusiast, but really just a southern Indiana farmer's son and engineering graduate from MIT.

Dr. Elizabeth Curtiss-Cabell, who wrote a monster dissertation under Barry's direction in implementing a host of epigenetics interventions in her special needs classroom and helped level

1 autism students off the spectrum altogether; Dr. Shannon Anderson, who with her father Jeff, helped design our first protocol and figured out ways to market it once our coaching business evolved; and to our amazing health and wellness coaches, Dr. Elaine Willerton, Dr. Jill Blackwell, Dr. Jeanine Ray, Dr. Jo Stone, and Dr. Marsha Ferrick, all clinical psychologists and our leaders of health coaching – an amazing team of outstanding, sensitive and experienced professionals.

A special word about Dr. Jo Stone, one of our coaches, who early on saw our vision and has never left the point of "being there" for me and for others, and who is always sacrificing and giving for the best and highest good; Dr. Rick Nida, Dr. Rich Hunter, both Ph.D. colleagues with me at Ohio University and real leaders in the healthcare business; and my dear long-time friend and colleague, Dr. Linda Larkey, Quigong and Tai Chi expert, who has written and led over 20 RO1 Research Grants through the National Institutes of Health, and also soft-spoken – and kept us focused.

Another former student and associate partner at IBM is Dale Harris who introduced our team to the IBM supercomputer, "Watson," currently able to do in minutes what it took us years to aggregate; Jacqueline Knight who brought her Madison Avenue talents to our marketing efforts; Dr. Gary Kreps, colleague and formerly a director of bioinformatics at NIH; Dr. Joe Veltman, geneticist and personal counselor; Dr. Craig Barton, engineer, statistician and mediator; Dr. Kimberly Kuden, who also has experienced the familial relationships and impacts of dementia; Dr. Rob Shah, financial genius and dear friend.

Jordana Gainsworth, advisor, with two doctorates in homeopathic healing; Bob Fox, our human resources advisor; Dr. Suzanne Peterson, a leadership guru, colleague, and co-author; Dr. Tom Littleton, former student, officer, ace pilot and problem-solver; Dr. Vanessa Ann Claus, who also understands the deep personal loss of family suffering with this disease; Dr. Linnea Rademaker, "storyteller" research; Dr. Heather Miller, our Institutional Review Board (IRB) expert; Dr. Debra Wood, our editor, proofreader, neuro-scientist and close friend.

Chuck Holman, our first investor and financial analyst; Nan Raden, another healer and close personal friend; Dr. Alan Castillo, who introduced us to the "cloud" where our capacious research could be kept; Dr. Anastasia Lande, another former student who persevered through her own health challenges and traveled to the Far East to better understand Ayurvedic medicine; Andrea Aristizabal, aka "Dayzee," a coach to the coaches and a healer of many years; and Jacqueline Tallarico who knows all there is to know about the brain.

And then there is Elle Coe; Bachelors in Applied Kinesiology and Exercise Physiology, Bachelors in Nursing and Masters/PhD is Psychology. An executive with one of the largest pharmaceutical organizations, Elle gave us a very grounded, pragmatic way to collaborate with pharma and healthcare. She saw what we were doing; she felt that different approaches were needed and believed in the possible outcomes. I am eternally grateful for discovering this amazing person!

Then there are the incredible editors from Story Monsters-our publisher, Linda Radke, our Project Manager, Patti Crane and our copy editor Ruthann Raitter. We simply could not have finished this project without them. Their deep experience and incredible skill-set gave us a "leg-up" for without it, we might still be writing, editing and then the research would have changed yet again. Thank you to all of you and thank you to Jerre Stead who introduced us to Linda and her amazing team of professionals.

And finally, but always in my heart, Felicitas Funke. Without her generous gifts and funds, we could not have been successful in getting this eBook to market.

As we said earlier, we wrote this eBook from a place of love and hope. We also think that when someone hears they have the early stages of dementia, they may be at a loss as to what to do next and where to go to seek the latest information. Now there is this eBook, and anyone and everyone can use this guide and this carefully curated, researched information to answer their questions and help them on their quest. With this eBook, you can be better informed and can communicate more effectively with your healthcare providers while making better decisions for yourself and your future. With this information, you can navigate the healthcare system, lessen the amount of anxiety you and your family may experience, and become a more active partner in the doctor-patient relationship and your own healing. In effect, you are creating a more patient-centered healthcare system.

As a final, personal note – I understand from the evidence that there is better than a 50/50 chance that I will develop some form of dementia as a result of my fall, suffering a traumatic brain injury (TBI). Had I not slipped that afternoon 40+ months ago, I perhaps would not have had the empathy and understanding of the dire situations many of us face, and I may not have had the drive to complete this project, go forth and put this eBook into the hands of many people who I hope might slow down their own cognitive decline, and those who think they might someday succumb. I'm one of those people, and I practice our **BEEMS** protocol every day. If you are reading this, then I hope you will read and follow our protocol as well.

We all need to listen to our makers, each other, our physicians and our higher power, and strive for a higher good and a purposeful life while we are on this planet. All the folks above did. I am immeasurably thankful and am a better person for having had them on my team, even if briefly.

Then there are other personal friends, all of whom started with me on this journey very early on. All four of these folks were Ph.D. students with me back in the 1970s and are still answering my calls: Dr. Roseanna Gaye Ross, Dr. Joe Chilberg, Dr. Robert Fischbach and Dr. Roger Desmond. They all read early drafts of the eBook, gave me some tough love and excellent feedback, and all did what friends are there to do. I am honored to call them my friends and they honor me by being there.

This was my chance to live a purposeful life, and I did.

Namaste,

Barry K. Spiker

LISTING OF ALL SOURCES EMBEDDED OR CITED

Preface

1. "Lifestyle Interventions Provide Maximum Memory Benefit When Combined; And May Offset Elevated Alzheimer's Risk Due to Genetics, Pollution". July 14, 2019. [website] https://www.prnewswire.com/news-releases/lifestyle-interventions-provide-maximum-memory-benefit-when-combined-and-may-offset-elevated-alzheimers-risk-due-to-genetics-pollution-300884442.html
2. Alzheimer's Disease International. (2018). World Alzheimer's report 2018 [website]. Retrieved from https://www.alz.co.uk/research/WorldAlzheimerReport2018.pdf

Introduction

3. Alzheimer's Association. (2019) Alzheimer's disease facts and figures. Retrieved from https://www.alz.org/media/Documents/alzheimers-facts-and-figures-2019-r.pdf
4. National Institute on Aging. (December 2017). Types of dementia. Retrieved from https://www.nia.nih.gov/health/alzheimers/basics
5. Sharma M, Raghuraman R, Sajikumar S. (2018). Epigenetics: The Panacea for Cognitive Decline? Retrieved from https://doi.org/10.18632/aging.101366

Influence from Your Environment

6. Dementia.org. (2015, July 2). Dementia from toxic substances [website]. Retrieved from https://www.dementia.org/dementia-from-poison-toxins

7. Sauer , A. (2018, September). Chronic Inflammation Linked to Dementia. Retrieved from https://www.alzheimers.net/chronic-inflammation-linked-to-dementia/

8. Newman, T. (2017, November). Could Inflammation in midlife predict dementia? Medical News Daily. Retrieved from https://www.medicalnewstoday.com/articles/319938.php

9. Riphagen, J. M., Gronenschild, E. H., Salat, D. H., Freeze, W. M., Ivanov, D., Clerx, L., ... & Jacobs, H. I. (2018). Shades of white: Diffusion properties of T1-and FLAIR-defined white matter signal abnormalities differ in stages from cognitively normal to dementia. *Neurobiology of Aging, 68*, 48–58. Retrieved from https://www.sciencedirect.com/science/article/pii/S0197458018301180?via%3Dihub

   a. Walker, K. A., Windham, B. G., Power, M. C., Hoogeveen, R. C., Folsom, A. R., Ballantyne, C. M., ... & Gottesman, R. F. (2018). The association of mid-to late-life systemic inflammation with white matter structure in older adults: The atherosclerosis risk in communities study. *Neurobiology of Aging, 68*, 26–33. Retrieved from https://www.sciencedirect.com/science/article/abs/pii/S0197458018301209?via%3Dihub

10. Sauer, A. (2019, April). Dementia and gut bacteria: New research shows link. Alzheimers.net. Retrieved from https://www.alzheimers.net/dementia-and-gut-bacteria-new-research-shows-link/

11. Akbari, E., Asemi, Z., Daneshvar Kakhaki, R., Bahmani, F., Kouchaki, E., Tamtaji, O. R., ... & Salami, M. (2016). Effect of probiotic supplementation on cognitive function and metabolic status in Alzheimer's disease: A randomized, double-blind and controlled trial. *Fron-

tiers in Aging Neuroscience, 8, 256. Retrieved from https://www.frontiersin.org/articles/10.3389/ fnagi.2016.00256/full

12. Bello, V. M. E., & Schultz, R. R. (2011). Prevalence of treatable and reversible dementias: A study in a dementia outpatient clinic. *Dementia & Neuropsychologia*, 5(1), 44–47. Retrieved from https:// www.ncbi.nlm.nih.gov/pmc/articles/PMC5619138/

13. Robertson, R. (2018, June). The gut-brain connection: How it works and the role of nutrition [website]. Healthline. Retrieved from https:// www.healthline.com/nutrition/gut-brain-connection

14. Mayo Clinic Staff. Dementia—Symptoms and Causes [website]. Retrieved from https:// www.mayoclinic.org/diseases-conditions/ dementia/symptoms-causes/syc-20352013

15. Beil, L. (2018, December).A gut-brain link for Parkinson's gets a closer look. Retrieved from https://www.sciencenews.org/article/ parkinsons-disease-gut-microbes-brain-link

What is Alzheimer's/Dementia/Cognitive Decline?

16. Alzheimer's Association. (2019). What Is mixed dementia? [website]. Alzheimer's Association. Retrieved from https://www.alz.org/ alzheimers-dementia/what-is-dementia/types-of-dementia/mixed-dementia.

17. James, B. D., Wilson, R. S., Boyle, P. A., Trojanowski, J. Q., Bennett, D. A., & Schneider, J. A. (2016). TDP-43 stage, mixed pathologies, and clinical Alzheimer's-type dementia. *Brain*, *139*(11), 2983–2993. Retrieved from https://www.ncbi.nlm.nih.gov/pmc/ articles/PMC5091047/

Long-Term Personal and Financial Costs

18. Alzheimer's Association. Testimony of Harry Johns, President, and CEO of the Alzheimer's Association. Retrieved from https://www.alz.org/documents/

national/submitted-testimony-050113.pdf

19. 60 Minutes, CBS News. (2018, August 12). Following a couple from diagnosis to the final stages of Alzheimer's. Retrieved from https://www.cbsnews.com/news/60-minutes-alzheimers-disease-following-a-couple-from-diagnosis-to-the-final-stages/

20. American Institute of Financial Gerontology [website]. Copyright 2019. Retrieved from. http://www.aifg.org/index.cfm.

21. MarketWatch (2015, November 10). Bank of America Merrill Lynch's director of financial gerontology Cyndi Hutchins named influencer in aging by PBS's Next Avenue. [website]. Retrieved from https://www.marketwatch.com/press-release/bank-of-america-merrill-lynchs-director-of-financial-gerontology-cyndi-hutchins-named-influencer-in-aging-by-pbss-next-avenue-2015-11-10

22. Us Against Alzheimer's [website]. (2019). Retrieved from https://www.usagainstalzheimers.org/

23. Next Avenue (2019). [website]. Retrievedfrom https://www.nextavenue.org/.

24. Zissimopoulos, J., Crimmins, E., & Clair, P. S. (2015). The value of delaying Alzheimer's disease onset. In *Forum for Health Economics and Policy* (Vol. 18, No. 1, pp. 25–39). Retrieved from https://europepmc.org/articles/pmc4851168

25. Awada, A. (2015). Early and late-onset Alzheimer's disease: What are the differences? *Journal of Neurosciences in Rural Practice*, 6(3), 455–456. Retrieved from https://www.ncbi.nlm.nih.gov/pmc/articles/PMC4481819/

26. Haaksma, M. L., Vilela, L. R., Marengoni, A., Calderón-Larrañaga, A., Leoutsakos, J. M. S., Rikkert, M. G. O., & Melis, R. J. (2017). Comorbidity and progression of late onset Alzheimer's disease: A systematic review.

PloS One, 12(5), e0177044. Retrieved from https://www.ncbi.nlm.nih.gov/pmc/articles/PMC5417646/

27. Duthie, A., Chew, D., & Soiza, R. L. (2011). Non-psychiatric comorbidity associated with Alzheimer's disease. *QJM: An International Journal of Medicine, 104*(11), 913–920. Retrieved from https://doi.org/10.1093/qjmed/hcr118

28. Garcez, M. L., Falchetti, A. C. B., Mina, F., & Budni, J. (2015). Alzheimer s disease associated with psychiatric comorbidities. *Anais da Academia Brasileira de Ciências, 87*(2), 1461–1473. Retrieved from https://dx.doi.org/10.1590/0001-3765201520140716

29. Snelling, S. (2014). Alzheimer's epidemic hits women hardest. Next Avenue [website]. Retrieved from https://www.nextavenue.org/alzheimers-epidemic-hits-women-hardest/

Prevention and the New Focus on Epigenetics

30. National Academies of Sciences, Engineering, and Medicine. (2017). *Preventing cognitive decline and dementia: A way forward.* Washington, DC: National Academies Press. Retrieved from https://www.ncbi.nlm.nih.gov/books/NBK436397/

31. Kane R. L., Butler M., Fink, H. A., Brasure, M., Davila, H., Desai, P., . . . Barclay T. (2017). Interventions to prevent age-related cognitive decline, mild cognitive impairment, and clinical Alzheimer's-type dementia. *Comparative Effectiveness* (Rev. No. 188). Retrieved from https://www.ncbi.nlm.nih.gov/books/NBK442425/

32. Fox, M. (2017, June). Not much can prevent Alzheimer's, but 3 common practices may help. Today Show, NBC News. Retrieved from https://www.today.com/series/one-small-thing/not-much-can-prevent-alzheimer-

s-3-things-may-help-t113051

33. Scott, P. (2018, April). The cheater's guide to beating Alzheimer's: New research and prevention breakthroughs. Parade Magazine Retrieved from https://parade.com/657576/paulaspencer/the-cheaters-guide-to-beating-alzheimers-new-research-and-prevention-breakthroughs/

34. Walsh, F. (2017, July). Nine lifestyle changes can reduce dementia risk, study says. *BBC news*. Retrieved from https://www.bbc.com/news/health-40655566

Epigenetics

35. Sharma, M., Raghuraman, R., Sajikumar, S. (2018). Epigenetics: The panacea for cognitive decline? *Aging, 10*(1), 1–2. Retrieved from https://doi.org/10.18632/aging.101366

36. Yehuda, R., Lehrner, A., & Bierer, L. M. (2018). The public reception of putative epigenetic mechanisms in the transgenerational effects of trauma. *Environmental Epigenetics*, 4(2), 1–7. Retrieved from https://doi.org/10.1093/eep/dvy018

37. Kirkpatrick, B. (2018, February 13). Muscles 'remember' previous exercise in the form of epigenetic tags on DNA [website]. Whatisepigenetics.com. Retrieved from https://www.whatisepigenetics.com/muscle-memory-epigenetic-exercise-tags/

38. Vickers, M. H. (2014). Early life nutrition, epigenetics and programming of later life disease. *Nutrients*, 6(6), 2165–2178. Retrieved from https://www.ncbi.nlm.nih.gov/pmc/articles/PMC4073141/

39. University of Illinois College of Agricultural, Consumer and Environmental Sciences. (2017, October 19). Maternal diet may program child for disease risk, but better nutrition later can change that. Retrieved from https://www.sciencedaily.com/

releases/2017/10/171019181846.htm.

40. Marx, G. & Chaim, G. (2012). The molecular basis of memory. *ACS Chemical Neuroscience, 3* (8), 633–642. Retrieved from https://pubs.acs.org/doi/full/10.1021/cn300097b

41. University of Bristol. (2013, March). Brain's 'molecular memory switch' identified. *ScienceDaily,* 28. Retrieved from https://www.sciencedaily.com/releases/2013/03/130328125226.htm

42. Lipton, B. (2015, September). The biology of belief. Retrieved from https://www.brucelipton.com/books/biology-of-belief

43. Cowell, I. (2019). Epigenetics–How does it work? . British Society for Cell Biology. Retrieved from https://bscb.org/learning-resources/softcell-e-learning/epigenetics-its-not-just-genes-that-make-us/

44. Weinhold B. (2006). Epigenetics: The science of change. *Environmental Health Perspectives, 114*(3), A160–A167. Retrieved from https://www.ncbi.nlm.nih.gov/pmc/articles/PMC1392256/

45. Barouki, R., Melén, E., Herceg, Z., Beckers, J., Chen, J., Karagas, M., … Nohara, K. "Epigenetics as a Mechanism Linking Developmental Exposures to Long-term Toxicity." Environment International, 114, 77–86. https://www.ncbi.nlm.nih.gov/pmc/articles/PMC5899930/.

The Most Important Studies of the BEEMS Protocol

46. Forks Over Knives. (2011). Directed by Lee Fulkerson, Written by Lee Fulkerson. Retrieved from https://en.wikipedia.org/wiki/Forks_Over_Knives

47. Campbell, Colin. "The China Study – The Movie." *Sustainable Media.* June 2017. http://sustainable.media/the-china-study-the-movie/.

Braak's Hypothesis

48. Rietdijk, C. D., Perez-Pardo, P., Garssen, J., van Wezel, R. J., & Kraneveld, A. D. (2017). Exploring Braak's hypothesis of Parkinson's disease. *Frontiers in Neurology*, *8*, 37. Retrieved from https://www.ncbi.nlm.nih.gov/pmc/articles/PMC5304413/

49. Lund University. (2014, October 13). Disputed theory on Parkinson's origin strengthened. *ScienceDaily.* Retrieved from https://www.sciencedaily.com/releases/2014/10/141013104153.htm

50. Kwon, D. Does Parkinson's Begin in the Gut? [website] (2018, May). *Scientific American*. Retrieved from https://www.scientificamerican.com/article/does-parkinsons-begin-in-the-gut/

51. Peter, I., Dubinsky, M., Bressman, S., Park, A., Lu, C., Chen, N., & Wang, A. (2018). Anti–tumor necrosis factor: Therapy and incidence of Parkinson disease among patients with inflammatory bowel disease. *JAMA Neurology*, *75*(8), 939–946. Retrieved from https://jamanetwork.com/journals/jamaneurology/article-abstract/2679038

52. Newman, T. (2019, February). Are we facing a Parkinson's pandemic? *Medical News Today.* Retrieved from https://www.medicalnewstoday.com/articles/324344.php?iacp

The Nun Study

53. Danner, D., Snowdon, D., Friesen, W. Positive emotions in early life and longevity: Findings from the Nun Study. University of Kentucky. Retrieved from https://www.apa.org/pubs/journals/releases/psp805804.pdf

54. Belluck, P. Nuns Offer Clues to Alzheimer's and Aging. (2001, May). NY Times. Retrieved

from https://www.nytimes.com/2001/05/07/us/ nuns-offer-clues-to-alzheimer-s-and-aging.html

55. Snowdon, D. A. (2003). Healthy aging and dementia: Findings from the Nun Study. *Annals of Internal Medicine, 139*(5), 450–454. Retrieved from https://www.ncbi.nlm.nih.gov/pubmed/12965975

PREDIVA Study (Dutch Prevention of Dementia by Intensive Vascular Care)

56. van Charante, E. P. M., Richard, E., Eurelings, L. S., van Dalen, J. W., Ligthart, S. A., Van Bussel, E. F., ... & van Gool, W. A. (2016). Effectiveness of a 6-year multidomain vascular care intervention to prevent dementia (preDIVA): A cluster-randomised controlled trial. *The Lancet, 388*(10046), 797–805. Retrieved from https://www.thelancet.com/journals/lancet/ article/PIIS0140-6736(16)30950-3/ fulltext#seccestitle10

The Finger Study

57. Kivipelto, M., Solomon, A., Ahtiluoto, S., Ngandu, T., Lehtisalo, J., Antikainen, R., ... & Lindström, J. (2013). The Finnish geriatric intervention study to prevent cognitive impairment and disability (FINGER): Study design and progress. *Alzheimer's & Dementia, 9*(6), 657–665. Retrieved from https://www.ncbi.nlm.nih.gov/pubmed/23332672

MAPT RCT (French Multidomain Alzheimer Preventive Trial--MAPT)

58. Vellas, B., Carrie, I., Gillette-Guyonnet, S., Touchon, J., Dantoine, T., Dartigues, J. F., ... & Bories, L. (2014). MAPT study: A multidomain approach for preventing Alzheimer's disease: Design and baseline data. *The*

Journal of Prevention of Alzheimer's Disease, 1(1), 13–. Retrieved from https://www.ncbi.nlm.nih.gov/pmc/articles/PMC4652787/

59. Richard, E., Jongstra, S., Soininen, H., Brayne, C., van Charante, E. P. M., Meiller, Y., ... & Ngandu, T. (2016). Healthy Ageing Through Internet Counselling in the Elderly: The HATICE randomised controlled trial for the prevention of cardiovascular disease and cognitive impairment. *BMJ Open, 6*(6), e010806. Retrieved from https://bmjopen.bmj.com/content/6/6/e010806

60. Livingston, G., Sommerlad, A., Orgeta, V., Costafreda, S. G., Huntley, J., Ames, D., ... & Cooper, C. (2017). Dementia prevention, intervention, and care. *The Lancet, 390*(10113), 2673–2734. Retrieved from https://www.ncbi.nlm.nih.gov/pubmed/28735855

The Pointer Study

61. Alzheimer's Association. (2019). U.S. POINTER: A lifestyle intervention trial to support brain health and prevent cognitive decline. Alzheimer's Association. Retrieved from https://alz.org/us-pointer/overview.asp

62. Anstey, K. J., Eramudugolla, R., Hosking, D. E., Lautenschlager, N. T., & Dixon, R. A. (2015). Bridging the translation gap: From dementia risk assessment to advice on risk reduction. *The Journal of Prevention of Alzheimer's Disease, 2*(3), 189. Retrieved from https://www.ncbi.nlm.nih.gov/pmc/articles/PMC4568745/

Breaking News—This Just In!

63. Caroll, L. (2019, July 14). Can Alzheimer's be stopped? Five lifestyle behaviors are key, new research suggests [website]. NBC News. Retrieved from https://www.nbcnews.com/health/aging/can-alzheimer-s-

be-stopped-five-lifestyle-behaviors-are-key-n1029441.

64. Lourida, I., Hannon, E., Littlejohns, T. J., Langa, K. M., Hyppönen, E., Kuźma, E., & Llewellyn, D. J. (2019). Association of lifestyle and genetic risk with incidence of dementia. *JAMA*, *322*(5), 430–437. Retrieved from https://www.sciencedaily.com/releases/2019/07/190714142509.htm.

65. Lourida I, Hannon E, Littlejohns TJ, et al. (2019). Association of Lifestyle and Genetic Risk With Incidence of Dementia. *JAMA*, Retrieved from https://jamanetwork.com/journals/jama/article-abstract/2738355.

66. Staff (2019, July 15). More proof that healthy lifestyle reduces cognitive impairment, dementia risk. Retrieved from https://www.healio.com/family-medicine/geriatric-medicine/news/online/%7B0803097d-ddcb-4795-9b51-d5a32acf952f%7D/more-proof-that-healthy-lifestyle-reduces-cognitive-impairment-dementia-risk.

67. Alzheimer's Association International. Lifestyle interventions provide maximum memory benefit when combined, may offset elevated Alzheimer's risk due to genetics, pollution . Retrieved from https://www.alz.org/aaic/releases_2019/sunLIFESTYLE-jul14.asp.

The BEEMS Approach—What You Can Do Now!

Body

68. National Institutes of Health. (2018, April). Lack of REM sleep linked to an increased risk of dementia [website]. Retrieved from https://www.nih.gov/news-events/lack-sleep-may-be-linked-risk-factor-alzheimers-disease.

69. Brzecka, A., Leszek, J., Ashraf, G. M., Ejma, M., Ávila-Rodriguez, M. F., Yarla, N. S., ... & Aliev, G. (2018). Sleep disorders associated with Alzheimer's disease: A perspective. *Frontiers in Neuroscience, 12*, 330. Retrieved from https://www.ncbi.nlm.nih.gov/pmc/articles/PMC5990625/.

70. Bhandari, T. (2017, July). Sleep, Alzheimer's link explained. Washington University of Medicine in St. Louis. Retrieved from https://medicine.wustl.edu/news/sleep-alzheimers-link-explained/.

71. Shi, L., Chen, S. J., Ma, M. Y., Bao, Y. P., Han, Y., Wang, Y. M., ... & Lu, L. (2018). Sleep disturbances increase the risk of dementia: A systematic review and meta-analysis. *Sleep Medicine Reviews, 40*, 4–16. Retrieved from https://doi.org/10.1016/j.smrv.2018.08.010.

Diet and Nutrition

72. Morris, M. C., Tangney, C. C., Wang, Y., Sacks, F. M., Bennett, D. A., & Aggarwal, N. T. (2015). MIND diet associated with reduced incidence of Alzheimer's disease. *Alzheimer's & Dementia: The Journal of the Alzheimer's Association, 11*(9), 1007–1014. Retrieved from https://www.ncbi.nlm.nih.gov/pmc/articles/PMC4532650/.

73. Pearson, K. (2017, July). What is the mind diet? Healthline.com. Retrieved from https://www.healthline.com/nutrition/mind-diet.

74. Gasior, M., Rogawski, M. A., & Hartman, A. L. (2006). Neuroprotective and disease-modifying effects of the ketogenic diet. *Behavioural Pharmacology, 17*(5–6), 431–439. Retrieved from https://www.ncbi.nlm.nih.gov/pmc/articles/PMC2367001/.

75. Barberger-Gateau, P., Raffaitin, C., Letenneur, L., Berr, C., Tzourio, C., Dartigues, J. F., & Alpérovitch, A. (2007). Dietary patterns and risk of dementia: The three-city cohort study. *Neurology, 69*(20), 1921–1930. Retrieved from https://www.ncbi.nlm.nih.gov/pubmed/17998483.

76. Yang, Y., Zhao, L. G., Wu, Q. J., Ma, X., & Xiang, Y. B.

(2015). Association between dietary fiber and lower risk of all-cause mortality: A meta-analysis of cohort studies. *American Journal of Epidemiology, 181*(2), 83–91. Retrieved from https://www.ncbi.nlm.nih.gov/pmc/articles/PMC6166337/.

77. University of California (2019). Why Is fiber good for you? University of California. Retrieved from https://www.ucsfbenioffchildrens.org/education/why_fiber_is_so_good_for_you/.

78. Rosenbloom, C. (2018, May). In large quantities, health foods can do more harm than good. *The Washington Post.* Retrieved from https://www.seattlepi.com/lifestyle/article/In-large-quantities-health-foods-can-do-more-12950939.php.

79. Rapaport, L. (2018, March). Drinking problems tied to higher risk. Reuters. Retrieved from https://www.reuters.com/article/us-health-dementia-alcohol/drinking-problems-tied-to-higher-risk-of-early-dementia-idUSKCN1GJ385.

80. Schwarzinger, M., Pollock, B. G., Hasan, O. S., Dufouil, C., Rehm, J., Baillot, S., … & Luchini, S. (2018). Contribution of alcohol use disorders to the burden of dementia in France 2008–13: A nationwide retrospective cohort study. *The Lancet Public Health, 3*(3), e124-e132. Retrieved from https://www.thelancet.com/journals/lanpub/article/PIIS2468-2667(18)30022-7/fulltext.

81. Reinagel, Monica. "Diet Soda and Dementia—What you Need to Know." *Scientific American.* August 2017. https://www.scientificamerican.com/article/diet-soda-and-dementia-what-you-need-to-know/.

82. Pase, Matthew P et al. "Sugar- and Artificially Sweetened Beverages and the Risks of Incident Stroke and Dementia: A Prospective Cohort Study." Stroke vol. 48,5 (2017): 1139-1146. https://

www.ncbi.nlm.nih.gov/pmc/articles/PMC5405737/.

83. Eskelinen M. H., Kivipelto M. (2010). Caffeine as a protective factor in dementia and Alzheimer's disease. *Journal of Alzheimer's Disease, 20*, S167–S174 S167. Retrieved from https://pdfs.semanticscholar.org/ee76/e52665ce5ffc9e6ba21ba1a58a5d059c59e1.pdf.

Supplements

84. St. Michael's Hospital. (2018, May). Study: Multivitamins, other common supplements have no health benefits. St. Michael's Hospital. Retrieved from https://www.sciencedaily.com/releases/2018/05/180528171511.htm.

85. McCleery, J., Abraham, R. P., Denton, D. A., Rutjes, A. W., Chong, L. Y., Al-Assaf, A. S., ... & Di Nisio, M. (2018). Vitamin and mineral supplementation for preventing dementia or delaying cognitive decline in people with mild cognitive impairment. *Cochrane Database of Systematic Reviews*, (11) Art. No.: CD011905. Retrieved from https://www.cochrane.org/CD011905/DEMENTIA_vitamin-and-mineral-supplementation-preventing-dementia-or-delaying-cognitive-decline-people-mild.

86. Sarker, M. R., & Franks, S. F. (2018). Efficacy of curcumin for age-associated cognitive decline: A narrative review of preclinical and clinical studies. *Geroscience,40*(2), 73–95. Retrieved from. https://www.ncbi.nlm.nih.gov/pmc/articles/PMC5964053/.

87. Enderami, A., Zarghami, M., & Darvishi-Khezri, H. (2018). The effects and potential mechanisms of folic acid on cognitive function: A comprehensive review. *Neurological Sciences, 39*(10), 1667–1675. Retrieved from https://www.ncbi.nlm.nih.gov/pubmed/29936555.

88. McCleery J, Abraham RP, Denton DA, Rutjes AWS, Chong L, Al-Assaf AS, Griffith DJ, Rafeeq S, Yaman H, Malik MA, Di Nisio M, Martínez G, Vernooij RWM, Tabet N. "Vitamin and Mineral Supplementation for

Preventing Dementia or Delaying Cognitive Decline in People with Mild Cognitive Impairment." *Cochrane Database of Systematic Reviews* 2018, Issue 11. Art. No.: CD011905. https://www.cochrane.org/CD011905/DEMENTIA_vitamin-and-mineral-supplementation-preventing-dementia-or-delaying-cognitive-decline-people-mild.

89. Kennedy, D. O. (2016). B vitamins and the brain: Mechanisms, dose and efficacy—a review. *Nutrients, 8*(2), 68–88. Retrieved from https://www.ncbi.nlm.nih.gov/pmc/articles/PMC4772032/.

90. Köbe T., Witte A. V., Schnelle, A, Lesemann, A., Fabian, S., Tesky, V. A., Pantel, J., Flöel, A. (2016). Omega-3 prevents decline in gray matter volume of the frontal, parietal and cingulate cortex in patients with mild cognitive impairments. *Neuroimage,131* 226–238. Retrieved from https://www.ncbi.nlm.nih.gov/pubmed/26433119.

Exercise

91. Xu, W., Wang, H. F., Wan, Y., Tan, C. C., Yu, J. T., & Tan, L. (2017). Leisure time physical activity and dementia risk: A dose-response meta-analysis of prospective studies. *BMJ Open, 7*(10), e014706. Retrieved from https://www.ncbi.nlm.nih.gov/pmc/articles/PMC5665289/.

92. Laurin, D., Verreault, R., Lindsay, J., MacPherson, K., & Rockwood, K. (2001). Physical activity and risk of cognitive impairment and dementia in elderly persons. *Archives of Neurology, 58*(3), 498–504. Retrieved from https://www.ncbi.nlm.nih.gov/pubmed/11255456.

93. Abbott, R. D., White, L. R., Ross, G. W., Masaki, K. H., Curb, J. D., & Petrovitch, H. (2004). Walking and dementia in physically capable elderly men. *JAMA, 292*(12), 1447–1453. Retrieved from https://www.ncbi.nlm.nih.gov/pubmed/15383515.

94. Neergaard, J. S., Dragsbæk, K., Hansen, H. B., Henriksen, K., Christiansen, C., & Karsdal, M. A. (2016). Late-life risk factors for all-cause dementia and

differential dementia diagnoses in women: A prospective cohort study. *Medicine, 95*(11), e3112. Retrieved from https://www.ncbi.nlm.nih.gov/pmc/articles/PMC4839938/.

95. Brasure, M., Desai, P., Davila, H., Nelson, V. A., Calvert, C., Jutkowitz, E., ... & McCarten, J. R. (2018). Physical activity interventions in preventing cognitive decline and Alzheimer-type dementia: A systematic review. *Annals of Internal Medicine, 168*(1), 30–38. Retrieved from https://www.ncbi.nlm.nih.gov/pubmed/29255839.

96. Sabia, S., Dugravot, A., Dartigues, J. F., Abell, J., Elbaz, A., Kivimäki, M., & Singh-Manoux, A. (2017). Physical activity, cognitive decline, and risk of dementia: 28 year follow-up of Whitehall II cohort study. *BMJ,357*, j2709. Retrieved from https://www.ncbi.nlm.nih.gov/pmc/articles/PMC5480222/.

97. Northey, J. M., Cherbuin, N., Pumpa, K. L., Smee, D. J., & Rattray, B. (2018). Exercise interventions for cognitive function in adults older than 50: a systematic review with meta-analysis. *British Journal of Sports Medicine, 52*(3), 154–160. Retrieved from. https://www.ncbi.nlm.nih.gov/pubmed/28438770.

98. Singh, M. A. F., Gates, N., Saigal, N., Wilson, G. C., Meiklejohn, J., Brodaty, H., ... & Baker, M. K. (2014). The Study of mental and resistance training (SMART) study—resistance training and/or cognitive training in mild cognitive impairment: A randomized, double-blind, double-sham controlled trial. *Journal of the American Medical Directors Association, 15*(12), 873–880. Retrieved from https://www.ncbi.nlm.nih.gov/pubmed/25444575.

99. Gates NJ, Vernooij RWM, Di Nisio M, Karim S, March E, Martínez G, Rutjes AWS. "Computerised Cognitive Training for Preventing Dementia in People with Mild Cognitive Impairment." Cochrane Database of Systematic Reviews 2019, Issue 3. Art. No.: CD012279. https://www.cochrane.org/CD012279/DEMENTIA_computerised-cognitive-training-preventing-dementia-people-mild-cognitive-impairment

100. Merzenith, Michael. "Does Scientific Evidence Show Brain Training Works?." CognitiveTrainingData.org. 2018. https://www.cognitivetrainingdata.org/the-controversy-does-brain-training-work/.

101. Tejal M. Shah, Michael Weinborn, Giuseppe Verdile, Hamid R. Sohrabi, Ralph N. Martins. "Enhancing Cognitive Functioning in Healthy Older Adults: a Systematic Review of the Clinical Significance of Commercially Available." *Neuropsychology Review,* 2017, Volume 27, Number 1. 2017. https://www.ncbi.nlm.nih.gov/pubmed/28092015.

102. Grothaus, Michael. "This Is The Only Type Of Brain Training That Works, According To Science." *Fast Company.* August 2017. https://www.fastcompany.com/40451692/this-is-the-only-type-of-brain-training-that-works-according-to-science.

103. Simons, D. J., Boot, W. R., Charness, N., Gathercole, S. E., Chabris, C. F., Hambrick, D. Z., & Stine-Morrow, E. A. L. (2016). "Do "Brain-Training" Programs Work?." *Psychological Science in the Public Interest,* 17(3), 103–186. https://www.ncbi.nlm.nih.gov/pubmed/27697851.

104. Yong, Ed. "The Weak Evidence Behind Brain-Training Games." *The Atlantic.* October 2016. https://www.theatlantic.com/science/archive/2016/10/the-weak-evidence-behind-brain-training-games/502559/.

Emotions

105. Institute for Health and Human Potential. (2019). What Is emotional intelligence? Retrieved from https://www.ihhp.com/meaning-of-emotional-intelligence.

106. Six Seconds Organization. Six Seconds EQ Network [website]. Retrieved from https://www.6seconds.org/.

107. Elementally EQ. Elementally EQ. Retrieved from http://www.elementallyeq.com/.

108. Dementia Care Central (2019). Dementia Care

Central [website]. Retrieved from https://www.dementiacarecentral.com/.

109. Guyoncourt, S. (2016, January).Chronic Stress Could Lead to Depression and Dementia, Scientists Warn [website]. The Independent. Retrieved from . Retrieved from https://www.independent.co.uk/lifestyle/health-and-families/health-news/chronic-stress-could-lead-to-depression-and-dementia-scientists-warn-a6831786.html.

110. Brigham Young University (2017, October 16). Stress might be just as unhealthy as junk food to digestive system: Study with mice shows stress causes digestive microorganisms to behave similar to how they act with high-fat diet. *ScienceDaily*. Retrieved from https://www.sciencedaily.com/releases/2017/10/171016142449.htm.

111. Khalsa, D. S. (2015). Stress, meditation, and Alzheimer's disease prevention: Where the evidence stands. *Journal of Alzheimer's Disease, 48*(1), 1–12. Retrieved from https://www.ncbi.nlm.nih.gov/pmc/articles/PMC4923750/.

112. University of Calgary. (2018, March).Is your stress changing my brain? Stress isn't just contagious; it alters the brain on a cellular level. *ScienceDaily*. Retrieved from https://www.sciencedaily.com/releases/2018/03/180308143212.htm.

113. Department of Community and Family Medicine. Duke Anxiety-Depression Scale (DUKE-AD). Duke University. Copyright 1994-2016. Retrieved from https://www.ncbi.nlm.nih.gov/pubmed/9085098.

114. Snell Jr, W. E., Gum, S., Shuck, R. L., Mosley, J. A., & Kite, T. L. (1995). The clinical anger scale: Preliminary reliability and validity. *Journal of Clinical Psychology, 51*(2), 215–226. Retrieved from https://www.ncbi.nlm.nih.gov/pubmed/7797645.

115. Beck Depression Inventory. Retrieved from https://www.ismanet.org/doctoryourspirit/pdfs/Beck-Depression-Inventory-BDI.pdf

116. Mayo Clinic Staff. Understanding uncontrollable crying or laughing. Mayo Clinic. 2019.Retrieved from https://www.mayoclinic.org/diseases-

conditions/pseudobulbar-affect/symptoms-causes/syc-20353737.

117. Mind Tools. How emotionally intelligent are you? Retrieved from https://www.mindtools.com/pages/article/ei-quiz.htm.

118. IHHP. Test your Emotional Intelligence with our Free EQ Quiz. Retrieved from https://www.ihhp.com/free-eq-quiz/.

Environment

119. Vlachokostas, C., Banias, G., Athanasiadis, A., Achillas, C., Akylas, V., & Moussiopoulos, N. (2014). Cense: A tool to assess combined exposure to environmental health stressors in urban areas. *Environment International, 63*, 1–10. Retrieved from https://www.ncbi.nlm.nih.gov/pubmed/24246237.

120. Public Health Ontario. Living near major traffic linked to higher risk of dementia. (2017, January) *ScienceDaily.* Retrieved from https://www.sciencedaily.com/releases/2017/01/170104192302.htm.

121. Chen, H., Kwong, J. C., Copes, R., Tu, K., Villeneuve, P. J., van Donkelaar, A., . . . Burnett, R. T. (2017). Living near major roads and the incidence of dementia, Parkinson's disease, and multiple sclerosis: A population-based cohort study. *The Lancet, 389*(10070), 718–726. Retrieved from https://www.thelancet.com/journals/lancet/article/PIIS0140-6736(16)32399-6/fulltext.

122. Moy, E., Garcia, M. C., Bastian, B., Rossen, L. M., Ingram, D. D., Faul, M., ... & Iademarco, M. F. (2017). Leading causes of death in nonmetropolitan and metropolitan areas—United States, 1999–2014. *MMWR Surveillance Summaries, 66*(1), 1–8. Retrieved from https://www.cdc.gov/mmwr/volumes/66/ss/ss6601a1.htm.

123. Chaix, B., Meline, J., Duncan, S., Jardinier, L., Perchoux, C., Vallee, J., ... & Kestens, Y. (2013). Neighborhood environments, mobility, and health: Towards a new generation of studies in environmental health

research. *Revue d'epidemiologie et de Sante Publique, 61,* S139–S145. Retrieved from https://www.ncbi.nlm.nih.gov/pubmed/23845204.

124. Economic Innovation Group. Website. Liu, J., Kelz, R. (2018, September). Types of hospitals in the US. JAMA Network. Retrieved from https://jamanetwork.com/journals/jama/fullarticle/2702148.

Mindfulness

125. Barbash, E. Mindfulness and being in the moment. (2018, January). Psychology Today. Retrieved from https://www.psychologytoday.com/us/blog/trauma-and-hope/201801/mindfulness-and-being-present-in-the-moment.

126. Selva, J. (2019, June). What is mindfulness? A psychologist explains. Positive Psychology Program. Retrieved from https://positivepsychologyprogram.com/what-is-mindfulness-definition/.

127. Mental Health Foundation. (2019). Look after Your Mental Health Using Mindfulness. Mental Health Foundation. Retrieved from https://www.mentalhealth.org.uk/your-mental-health/looking-after-your-mental-health.

128. NHS. (2019). Mindfulness: It can be easy to rush through life without stopping to notice much. NHS. Retrieved from https://www.nhs.uk/conditions/stress-anxiety-depression/mindfulness/.

129. The Science Behind Mindfulness Meditation. Retrieved from https://www.youtube.com/watch?v=VTAOj8FfCvs.

130. Why Mindfulness Is a Superpower: An Animation. Retrieved from https://www.youtube.com/watch?v=w6T02g5hnT4.

131. Happify. (2019). Happify is the Single Destination for Effective, Evidence-based Solutions for Better Emotional Health and Wellbeing in the 21st Century. Retrieved from https://www.happify.com/.

132. Bornstein, R. F. (2015). Personality assessment in the

diagnostic manuals: On mindfulness, multiple methods, and test score discontinuities. *Journal of Personality Assessment, 97*(5), 446–455. Retrieved from. https://www.ncbi.nlm.nih.gov/pmc/articles/PMC4545313/.

133. Larouche, E., Hudon, C., & Goulet, S. (2015). Potential benefits of mindfulness-based interventions in mild cognitive impairment and Alzheimer's disease: An interdisciplinary perspective. *Behavioural Brain Research, 276*, 199–212. Retrieved from https://www.ncbi.nlm.nih.gov/pubmed/24893317.

134. Aboutmeditation.com. (2019).Meditation 101: A beginner's guide. Retrieved from https://aboutmeditation.com/temp-store/.

Spirituality

135. Carr, T. J., Hicks-Moore, S., & Montgomery, P. (2011). What's so big about the little things: A phenomenological inquiry into the meaning of spiritual care in dementia. *Dementia, 10*(3), 399–414. Retrieved from https://journals.sagepub.com/doi/10.1177/1471301211408122.

136. Aldwin, C. M., Park, C. L., Jeong, Y. J. & Nath, R. (2014). Different pathways between religiousness spirituality and health a self-regulation perspective. *Psychology of Religion and Spirituality, 6*(1), 9–21. Retrieved from https://psycnet.apa.org/record/2013-44401-001.

137. Beuscher, L., & Beck, C. (2008). A literature review of spirituality in coping with early-stage Alzheimer's disease. *Journal of Clinical Nursing, 17*(5a), 88–97. Retrieved from https://onlinelibrary.wiley.com/doi/full/10.1111/j.1365-2702.2007.02126.x.

138. Dalby, P., Sperlinger, D. J., & Boddington, S. (2012). The lived experience of spirituality and dementia in older people living with mild to moderate dementia. *Dementia, 11*(1), 75–94. Retrieved from https://journals.sagepub.com/doi/10.1177/1471301211416608.

139. Boyle, P. A., Buchman, A. S., Barnes, L. L., & Bennett,

D. A. (2010). Effect of a purpose in life on risk of incident Alzheimer disease and mild cognitive impairment in community-dwelling older persons. *Archives of General Psychiatry, 67*(3), 304–310. Retrieved from https://www.ncbi.nlm.nih.gov/pmc/articles/PMC2897172/.

140. Bryden, C. (2002). A person-centred approach to counselling, psychotherapy and rehabilitation of people diagnosed with dementia in the early stages. *Dementia, 1*(2), 141–156. Retrieved from https://journals.sagepub.com/doi/10.1177/147130120200100203.

141. Ng, S. M., Yau, J. K., Chan, C. L., Chan, C. H., & Ho, D. Y. (2005). The measurement of body-mind-spirit well-being: Toward multidimensionality and transcultural applicability. *Social Work in Health Care, 41*(1), 33–52. Retrieved from https://www.tandfonline.com/doi/abs/10.1300/J010v41n01_03.

142. FACIT.org. Retrieved from https://www.facit.org/FACITOrg/Questionnaires.

143. S. M. Ng RSW, RCMPa, Josephine K. Y. Yau MPhil, BSSca, Cecilia L. W. Chan PhDa, Celia H. Y. Chan MSW, BSSc, RSWa & David Y. F. "The Measurement of Body-Mind-Spirit Well-Being: Toward Multidimensionality and Transcultural Applicability" in Social Work in Health Care". Ho PhDa pages 33-52 Volume 41, Issue 1, 2005. https://www.ncbi.nlm.nih.gov/pubmed/16048855.

Alternative Therapies and Dementia

144. Yakimicki, M. L., Edwards, N. E., Richards, E., & Beck, A. M. (2019). Animal-assisted intervention and dementia: A systematic review. *Clinical Nursing Research, 28*(1), 9–29. Retrieved from https://journals.sagepub.com/doi/10.1177/1054773818756987.

145. Wood, W., Fields, B., Rose, M., & McLure, M. (2017). Animal-assisted therapies and dementia: A systematic mapping review using the lived environment

life quality (LELQ) model. *American Journal of Occupational Therapy, 71*(5), 1–10. Retrieved from https://ajot.aota.org/article.aspx?articleid=2645783.

146. Sarah C. Slayton, Jeanne D'Archer & Frances Kaplan. "Outcome Studies on the Efficacy of Art Therapy: A Review of Findings." Art Therapy, 27:3, (2010) 108-118. https://www.arttherapy.org/upload/outcomes.pdf.

147. Ellen Greene Stewart. "Art Therapy and Neuroscience Blend: Working with Patients Who Have Dementia." Art Therapy, 21:3, 148-155 (2004). https://eric.ed.gov/?id=EJ682599.

148. Dementia Dynamics. "Painting in Twilight: An Artist's Escape from Alzheimer's." October 2010. https://dementiadynamics.com/painting-in-twilight-an-artists-escape-from-alzheimers/.

149. ALZOC.org. "Memories in the Making: Using art as a Communication Tool for People with Memory Loss." ALZOC.org. 2019. https://www.alzoc.org/memories-in-the-making/.

150. Nimer, J., & Lundahl, B. (2007). Animal-assisted therapy: A meta-analysis. *Anthrozoös, 20*(3), 225–238. Retrieved from https://www.tandfonline.com/doi/abs/10.2752/089279307X224773.

151. Creagan, E. T., Bauer, B. A., Thomley, B. S., & Borg, J. M. (2015). Animal-assisted therapy at Mayo Clinic: The time is now. *Complementary therapies in clinical practice, 21*(2), 101–104. Retrieved from https://www.sciencedirect.com/science/article/pii/S1744388115000249?via%3Dihub.

152. American Dance Therapy Association. (2019). What is Dance/Movement Therapy? [website]. Retrieved from https://adta.org/2014/11/08/what-is-dancemovement-therapy/.

153. Hanford, N., & Figueiro, M. (2013). Light therapy and Alzheimer's disease and related dementia: Past, present, and future. *Journal of Alzheimer's Disease, 33*(4), 913–922. Retrieved from https://www.ncbi.nlm.nih.gov/pmc/articles/PMC3553247/.

154. Figueiro, M. G. (2017). Light, sleep and circadian rhythms in older adults with Alzheimer's disease and related dementias. *Neurodegenerative disease management, 7*(2), 119–145. Retrieved from https://www.ncbi.nlm.nih.gov/pmc/articles/PMC5836917/.

155. Rotolo, Candace. (2019). Man in nursing home reacts to hearing music from his era. . Retrieved from https://www.agingcare.com/articles/man-nursing-home-reacts-hearing-music-from-era-150484.htm.

156. Svansdottir, H. B., & Snaedal, J. (2006). Music therapy in moderate and severe dementia of Alzheimer's type: A case-control study. *International Psychogeriatrics, 18*(4), 613–621. Retrieved from https://www.ncbi.nlm.nih.gov/pubmed/16618375.

157. Landis-Shack, N., Heinz, A. J., & Bonn-Miller, M. O. (2017). Music therapy for posttraumatic stress in adults: A theoretical review. *Psychomusicology: Music, Mind, and Brain, 27*(4), 334–342. Retrieved from https://www.ncbi.nlm.nih.gov/pmc/articles/PMC5744879/.

158. John Boehner and Bill Weld to join Acreage Board of Directors (April 2018). Retrieved from https://www.acreageholdings.com/newsroom/2018/8/9/john-boehner-and-bill-weld-to-join-acreage-board-of-directors.

159. National Institutes of Health. NIH research on marijuana and cannabinoids [website]. Retrieved from https://www.drugabuse.gov/drugs-abuse/marijuana/nih-research-marijuana-cannabinoids.

160. National Academies of Sciences, Engineering, and Medicine. (2017, January). Nearly 100 Conclusions on the Health Effects of Marijuana and Cannabis-Derived Products Presented in New Report; One of the Most Comprehensive Studies of Recent Research on Health Effects of Recreational and Therapeutic Use of Cannabis and Cannabis-Derived Products. Retrieved from https://www8.nationalacademies.org/onpinews/newsitem.aspx?RecordID=24625.

161. National Academies of Sciences, Engineer-

ing, and Medicine. (2017). *The health effects of cannabis and cannabinoids: The current state of evidence and recommendations for research*. Washington, DC: The National Academies Press. Retrieved from https://www.nap.edu/catalog/24625/the-health-effects-of-cannabis-and-cannabinoids-the-current-state.

162. University of Bonn. (2017, May 8). Cannabis reverses aging processes in the brain, study suggests: Researchers restore the memory performance of Methuselah mice to a juvenile stage. *ScienceDaily*. Retrieved from https://www.sciencedaily.com/releases/2017/05/170508112400.htm.

163. Santibanez, R. A., Sepehry, A. A., & Hsiung, G. Y. R. (2017). Cannabis and Alzheimer's disease: A systematic review of the evidence. *Alzheimer's & Dementia: The Journal of the Alzheimer's Association, 13*(7), 614. Retrieved from https://www.sciencedirect.com/science/article/pii/S155252601730907X.

164. Cao, C., Li, Y., Liu, H., Bai, G., Mayl, J., Lin, X., … & Cai, J. (2014). The potential therapeutic effects of THC on Alzheimer's disease. *Journal of Alzheimer's Disease, 42*(3), 973–984. Retrieved from https://www.ncbi.nlm.nih.gov/pubmed/25024327.

165. Aso, E., & Ferrer, I. (2014). Cannabinoids for treatment of Alzheimer's disease: Moving toward the clinic. *Frontiers in Pharmacology, 5*, 37. 1–11. Retrieved from https://www.ncbi.nlm.nih.gov/pmc/articles/PMC3942876/

166. Karl, T., Garner, B., & Cheng, D. (2017). The therapeutic potential of the phytocannabinoid cannabidiol for Alzheimer's disease. *Behavioural Pharmacology, 28*(2/3), 142–160. Retrieved from https://www.ncbi.nlm.nih.gov/pubmed/27471947.

167. Boehnke, K. F., Litinas, E., & Clauw, D. J. (2016). Medical cannabis use is associated with decreased opiate medication use in a retrospective cross-sectional survey of patients with chronic pain. *Journal of Pain, 17*(6), 739–744. Retrieved from https://www.ncbi.nlm.nih.gov/pubmed/27001005.

168. United Patients Group. (2017, March). Undeniable

evidence: Cannabis, Alzheimer's and dementia. Retrieved from https://unitedpatientsgroup.com/blog/2017/03/15/undeniable-evidence-cannabis-alzheimers-and-dementia/.

Traumatic Brain Injury and Its Connections to Dementia

169. Centers for Disease Control and Prevention. Retrieved from https://www.cdc.gov/traumaticbraininjury/index.html.

170. Snell, W. E., Jr., Gum, S., Shuck, R. L., Mosley, J. A., & Kite, T. L. (1995). The clinical anger scale: Preliminary reliability and validity. *Journal of Clinical Psychology*, 51(2), 215-226. https://www.psytoolkit.org/survey-library/anger-cas.html#_introduction.

171. Stocchetti, N., & Zanier, E. R. (2016). Chronic impact of traumatic brain injury on outcome and quality of life: A narrative review. *Critical Care*, *20*(1), 148. Retrieved from https://ccforum.biomedcentral.com/articles/10.1186/s13054-016-1318-1

172. Marshall, T., & Henricks, C. (2017). The next generation in brain recovery and neuroregeneration. *Journal of American Physicians and Surgeons*, 22(2), 44–47. Retrieved from https://www.jpands.org/vol22no2/henricks.pdf.

173. Brazier, Y. (2016, September). What is hyperbaric oxygen therapy good for? Medical News Today. Retrieved from https://www.medicalnewstoday.com/articles/313155.php.

174. Neil B. Hampson, James Holm. "Letter re: Hyperbaric oxygen: B-Level evidence in mild traumatic brain injury clinical trials." *Neurology* Aug 2017, 89 (7) 750. https://n.neurology.org/content/89/7/750.2.

175. Shively, S., Scher, A. I., Perl, D. P., & Diaz-Arrastia, R. (2012). Dementia resulting from traumatic brain injury: What is the pathology? *Archives of Neurology*, *69*(10), 1245–1251. Retrieved from https://www.ncbi.nlm.nih.gov/pmc/articles/PMC3716376/.

176. Paddock, C. Even Mild TBI Might Raise Dementia

Risk . Medical News Today. May 2018. Retrieved from https://www.medicalnewstoday.com/articles/321740.php.

177. Barnes, D. E., Byers, A. L., Gardner, R. C., Seal, K. H., Boscardin, W. J., & Yaffe, K. (2018). Association of mild traumatic brain injury with and without loss of consciousness with dementia in US military veterans. *JAMA Neurology, 75*(9), 1055–1061. Retrieved from https://jamanetwork.com/journals/jamaneurology/article-abstract/2679879.

178. Fleminger, S., Oliver, D. L., Lovestone, S., Rabe-Hesketh, S., & Giora, A. (2003). Head injury as a risk factor for Alzheimer's disease: The evidence 10 years on; a partial replication. *Journal of Neurology, Neurosurgery & Psychiatry, 74*(7), 857–862. Retrieved from https://www.ncbi.nlm.nih.gov/pmc/articles/PMC1738550/.

179. Z. Guo, L.A. Cupples, A. Kurz, S.H. Auerbach, L. Volicer, H. Chui, R.C. Green, A.D. Sadovnick, R. Duara, C. DeCarli, K. Johnson, R.C. Go, J.H. Growdon, Jonathan L. Haines, W.A. Kukull, L.A. Farrer. "Head injury and the risk of AD in the MIRAGE study." *Neurology* Mar 2000, 54 (6) 1316-1323. https://n.neurology.org/content/54/6/1316.long.

180. Li, Y., Li, Y., Li, X., Zhang, S., Zhao, J., Zhu, X., & Tian, G. (2017). Head injury as a risk factor for dementia and Alzheimer's disease: A systematic review and meta-analysis of 32 observational studies. *PloS One, 12*(1), e0169650. Retrieved from https://www.ncbi.nlm.nih.gov/pmc/articles/PMC5221805/.

181. National Council on Aging. National Falls Prevention Resource Center. Retrieved from https://www.ncoa.org/center-for-healthy-aging/falls-resource-center/

182. National Council on Aging. Evidence-based falls prevention programs. Retrieved from https://www.ncoa.org/healthy-aging/falls-prevention/falls-prevention-programs-for-older-adults-2/.

183. Fang, W. L., Jiang, M. J., Gu, B. B., Wei, Y. M., Fan, S. N.,

Liao, W., ... & Xiao, S. H. (2018). Tooth loss as a risk factor for dementia: Systematic review and meta-analysis of 21 observational studies. *BMC Psychiatry*, *18*(1), 345. Retrieved from https://www.ncbi.nlm.nih.gov/pmc/articles/PMC6195976/.

184. Goldstein, J. YEAR. Fighting the TBI wars : New alternatives for TBI survivors. Retrieved from https://www.brainline.org/story/fighting-tbi-wars-new-alternatives-tbi-survivors.

Tests to Assess an Individual's Cognitive Decline

185. Soo Borson. Mini-Cog. Retrieved from https://mini-cog.com/.

186. The Montreal Cognitive Assessment. Retrieved from https://www.mocatest.org/the-moca-test/.

187. SAGE: A test to detect signs of Alzheimer's and dementia. Retrieved from https://wexnermedical.osu.edu/brain-spine-neuro/memory-disorders/sage

Epigenesis Corporation

188. Zissimopoulos, Julie et al. "The Value of Delaying Alzheimer's Disease Onset." Forum for health economics & policy vol. 18,1 (2014): 25-39. https://www.ncbi.nlm.nih.gov/pmc/articles/PMC4851168/.

189. Epigenesis Corporation Homepage. Retrieved from https://www.epigenesiscorp.com

190. Preventing Alzheimer's and Other Dementias NOW Website. Retrieved from https://www.preventingalzheimers.com

191. Matthew Baumgart, Heather M. Snyder, Maria C. Carrillo, Sam Fazioc, Hye Kim, Harry Johns.

192. Summary of the evidence on modifiable risk factors for cognitive decline and dementia: A population-based perspective. Retrieved from https://www.alzheimersanddementia.com/article/S1552-5260(15)00197-1/pdf.

193. Ngandu, T., Lehtisalo, J., Solomon, A., Levälahti, E.,

Ahtiluoto, S., Antikainen, R., ... & Lindström, J. (2015). A 2 year multidomain intervention of diet, exercise, cognitive training, and vascular risk monitoring versus control to prevent cognitive decline in at-risk elderly people (FINGER): A randomised controlled trial. *The Lancet, 385*(9984), 2255–2263. Retrieved from https://www.thelancet.com/journals/lancet/article/PIIS0140-6736(15)60461-5/fulltext#articleInformation.

194. Being Patient. (2017, October). Inside the FINGER Study: Hard evidence shows how diet, exercise and mind games might make or break a dementia diagnosis. Retrieved from https://www.beingpatient.com/finger-study/.

195. Clinical Trials.gov. US Study to Protect Brain Health Through Lifestyle Intervention to Reduce Risk (POINTER). Retrieved from https://clinicaltrials.gov/ct2/show/NCT03688126.

196. Point of Contact: Kit, brian. Framingham Heart Study. Retrieved from http://www.framinghamheartstudy.org/.

197. Peterson, Suzanne & Spiker, Barry. (2005). Establishing the positive contributory value of older workers: A positive psychology perspective. organizational dynamics. 34. 153–167. Retrieved from https://www.researchgate.net/publication/232427905_Establishing_the_Positive_Contributory_Allowed Value_of_Older_Workers_A_Positive_Psychology_Perspective.

The Platforms of Behavioral Change

198. Roche, N., & Bourbeau, J. (2016). Health coaching: another component of personalized medicine for patients with chronic obstructive pulmonary disease. *American Journal of Respiratory and Critical Care Medicine, 194*(6). Retrieved from. https://www.atsjournals.org/doi/10.1164/rccm.201604-0696ED.

199. Wolever, R. Q., Simmons, L. A., Sforzo, G. A., Dill, D.,

Kaye, M., Bechard, E. M., ... & Yang, N. (2013). A systematic review of the literature on health and wellness coaching: defining a key behavioral intervention in healthcare. *Global advances in health and medicine*, *2*(4), 38–57. Retrieved from https://www.ncbi.nlm.nih.gov/pmc/articles/PMC3833550/.

200. Substance Abuse and Mental Health Services Administration. National Helpline. Retrieved from https://www.samhsa.gov/find-help/national-helpline

201. US Department of Health and Human Services. (2007). *Alcohol alert.* (Report No. 71), Retrieved from https://pubs.niaaa.nih.gov/publications/aa71/aa71.htm.

202. Wagener, D. (2019, June). What is the success rate of AA? Retrieved from https://americanaddictioncenters.org/rehab-guide/12-step/whats-the-success-rate-of-aa.

203. National Center for Chronic Disease Prevention and Health Promotion. (2011). Quitting smoking among adults—United States, 2001—2010. *MMWR, 60*(44), 1513–1519. Retrieved from https://www.cdc.gov/mmwr/preview/mmwrhtml/mm6044a2.htm.

204. Psychology Today. Solution-focused brief therapy . Retrieved from https://www.psychologytoday.com/us/therapy-types/solution-focused-brief-therapy.

205. Gaudiano, B. A. (2008). Cognitive-behavioural therapies: Achievements and challenges. *Evidence-Based Mental Health*, *11*(1), 5–7. Retrieved from https://www.ncbi.nlm.nih.gov/pmc/articles/PMC3673298/.

206. Grohol, J. (2018, October). An overview of dialectical behavior therapy. Retrieved from https://psychcentral.com/lib/an-overview-of-dialectical-behavior-therapy/.

207. The Empowerment Partnership with Dr. Matt. Retrieved from http://www.nlp.com/what-is-nlp/.

208. Mills, T. What is natural language processing and what is it used for? Forbes Technology Council,

Forbes Magazine. Retrieved from https://www.forbes.com/sites/forbestechcouncil/2018/07/02/what-is-natural-language-processing-and-what-is-it-used-for/#493d48a65d71.

209. Williams, R. Rob Williams Shares about PSYCH-K . Retrieved from https://subconsciouschange.com/success-stories/supporters-and-science/rob-williams-m-a/.

210. Psych-K Centre International. Frequently Asked Questions . Retrieved from https://psych-k.com/frequently-asked-questions/.

211. Goyer, A.(2015). Juggling life, work, and caregiving. Retrieved from https://www.amazon.com/Juggling-Life-Work-Caregiving-Goyer/dp/1634251636.

212. MetLife. The MetLife study of caregiving costs to working caregivers. Retrieved from https://www.caregiving.org/wp-content/uploads/2011/06/mmi-caregiving-costs-working-caregivers.pdf.

213. Stanford study focuses on effects of family caregiving for patients with Alzheimer's disease and dementia. Retrieved from https://med.stanford.edu/news/all-news/2002/05/stanford-study-focuses-on-effects-of-family-caregiving-for-patients-with-alzheimers-disease-dementia.html.

214. Sheets, D. J., Black, K., & Kaye, L. W. (2014). Who cares for caregivers? Evidence-based approaches to family support. *Journal of Gerontological Social Work*, *57*(6-7), 525-530. Retrieved from, https://www.tandfonline.com/doi/full/10.1080/01634372.2014.920606.

215. Newton-Small, J. (2019, February). A growing American crisis: Who will care for the baby boomers? *Time Magazine*. Retrieved from. https://time.com/5529152/elderly-caregiving-baby-boomers-unpaid-caregivers-crisis/.

216. National Alliance for Caregiving. [website]. Retrieved from https://www.caregiving.org/resources/.

217. Alzheimer's Foundation of America. Retrieved from https://alzfdn.org/
218. National Council on Aging. Retrieved from https://www.ncoa.org/
219. Caregiving Organization. Retrieved from https://www.caregiving.org/
220. Caregiver Action Network. Retrieved from https://caregiveraction.org/
221. National Family Caregivers Association. Retrieved from https://www.caringcommunity.org/helpful-resources/models-research/national-family-caregivers-association-nfca/.
222. American Association of Retired People. Caregiving Innovation frontiers. Retrieved from https://www.aarp.org/content/dam/aarp/home-and-family/personal-technology/2017/08/caregiving-innovation-frontiers-2017-aarp.pdf.
223. American Society on Aging. Retrieved from 25 Organizations that Take Care of Caregivers. https://www.asaging.org/blog/25-organizations-take-care-caregivers.

Dementia's Impact on All Organizations

224. The Impact of Caregivers in the Workplace. (2017, June). Retrieved from https://www.dhs.wisconsin.gov/dementia/dfe-toolkit-impact.htm.
225. Fuller, J., & Raman, M. (2019). The caring company. *Harvard Business School*, 16. Retrieved from https://www.hbs.edu/managing-the-future-of-work/Documents/The_Caring_Company.pdf.
226. Shoptaugh, C. F., Phelps, J. A., & Visio, M. E. (2004). Employee eldercare responsibilities: Should organizations care? *Journal of Business and Psychology, 19*(2), 179–196. Retrieved from https://link.springer.com/article/10.1007%2Fs10869-004-0547-5.
227. Bagchi, A. Tomorrow is promised to no one. Retrieved from https://www.yourquote.in/arijit-bagchi-gf5e/quotes/time-

passes-so-quickly-you-don-t-even-notice-untill-it-show-g9ise.

<u>Acknowledgments</u>

228. Farmers Tribute: So God Made a Farmer. Paul Harvey . Retrieved from https://youtu.be/QuzhwkaNC40.

9 798692 038050